To the seven founders of La Leche League International, who courageously changed the world to make it possible for us to mother our children through breastfeeding, and to the Breastfeeding After Reduction (BFAR) and Mothers Overcoming Breastfeeding Issues (MOBI) online communities, who bravely explore ways to increase their milk production, often thinking outside the box and creating new ways to make more milk for their babies.

"This book is a great resource for all mothers, not just ones with milk supply issues. I was reassured that I was doing the right thing and found all the answers to my questions. It's like having a personal lactation consultant guiding me along."

—Ann Buskey, mother of two breastfed babies

"Even professionals with years of experience will learn new things. I predict this book will soon be known as the 'milk supply bible.'"

—Kathleen Kendall-Tackett, Ph.D., IBCLC,
coauthor of *Breastfeeding Made Simple*

"No one knows more about making more milk than Diana West and Lisa Marasco. Their combined wisdom and experience shine through in this much-needed resource."

—Nancy Mohrbacher, IBCLC,
coauthor of *The Breastfeeding Answer Book* and
Breastfeeding Made Simple

"Finally, a guidebook for mothers navigating the milk supply waters!"

—Jan Ellen Brown, RDH, IBCLC,
coauthor of *25 Things Every Nursing Mother Should Know*

"A scientifically studied book written with a mother's heart. It's an excellent addition to a professional's reference library or a mother's bedside table."

—Ann Perrine, M.D., La Leche League Leader

"This book shares its abundant wisdom with the warmth and support of a knowledgeable friend. It gently guides mothers along the difficult journey to find solutions to their milk supply issues."

—Laura Larocca, La Leche League Leader and
mother of five breastfed children

The Breastfeeding Mother's Guide to

Making
More Milk

Diana West, IBCLC, and
Lisa Marasco, M.A., IBCLC

New York Chicago San Francisco Lisbon London Madrid Mexico City
Milan New Delhi San Juan Seoul Singapore Sydney Toronto

The McGraw·Hill Companies

Library of Congress Cataloging-in-Publication Data

West, Diana (Diana Lynn).
  The breastfeeding mother's guide to making more milk / Diana West and Lisa Marasco.
     p.   cm.
  Includes bibliographical references and index.
  ISBN-13: 978-0-07-159857-6 (alk. paper)
  ISBN-10: 0-07-159857-X (alk. paper)
  1. Breast milk.   2. Breastfeeding.   I. Marasco, Lisa.   II. Title.

  QP246.W47   2009
  649'.33—dc22   2008013813

8 9 10 11 12 13 14 15 16 17 18 19 20 21 22   DOC/DOC 1 9 8 7 6 5 4 3 2 1

ISBN 978-0-07-159857-6
MHID   0-07-159857-X

Cartoon on page 3 is copyright © Hale Publishing, LP, from "Is He Biting Again?" by Neil Matterson, and used with permission.
Illustration on page 5 is copyright © Medela AG, Switzerland, 2006, and used with permission.
"The Murphy Maneuver" on page 92 by James Murphy, M.D., is used with permission.
Photo on page 104 is copyright © Diane Lewis Photography and used with permission.
"Power Pumping" on page 163 by Catherine Watson Genna, B.S., IBCLC, is used with permission.
Interior illustrations on pages 110 and 113 by Taina Litwak, CMI

McGraw-Hill books are available at special quantity discounts to use as premiums and sales promotions or for use in corporate training programs. To contact a representative, please visit the Contact Us pages at www.mhprofessional.com.

This book is offered for educational and informational purposes only and should not be construed as personal medical advice. The information herein is not intended to diagnose or treat any medical condition. It is important to inform both your and your baby's physicians of your issues and concerns with low milk production so that both your and your baby's health can be followed closely by a qualified health care professional.

This book is printed on acid-free paper.

Contents

Foreword

When women get together and start swapping stories of the days when their babies were small and the subject of breastfeeding comes up, chances are at least one woman will say, "I couldn't make enough (or my doctor said I didn't have enough) milk, so I had to quit nursing." If the subject changes quickly, no one gets to hear the sadness behind those words or the questions that could be asked: "What happened? Did anyone give you a reason?" That's where this book comes in. When there's another baby on the horizon, that same woman will grab this book right out of your hand. She wants answers, and *The Breastfeeding Mother's Guide to Making More Milk* has them. She needs to know she didn't fail; the problem was that the answers weren't there for her before. And there is plenty she can do to make more milk for the next baby.

Breastfeeding problems of one sort or another have been around forever, but good help for the complicated problems is still evolving. Many doctors, nurses, and even midwives haven't yet heard of all the advances in the field of lactation, so women are still being told they can't make more milk or shouldn't even consider breastfeeding at all. One example close to my heart is how mothers of babies with Down syndrome are often discouraged from breastfeeding. When I gave birth to Stephen eighteen years ago, his pediatrician thought I was being "heroic" for sticking with it through four long weeks of weight loss before he turned the corner and learned how to suck without hurting me. Until our culture is convinced that breastfeeding and breast milk make a difference, it is likely that this attitude will continue.

The first wave of breastfeeding help came from the founding mothers of La Leche League in 1956. The second wave, which resulted in the field of lactation science, began with passionate La Leche League Leaders who helped one mother and then another and then another, moving past the "easy" cases to the ones that needed more time and attention, more research, and more persistence. These are the cases you'll read about in this book, and you'll see the work of these pioneers listed in the References.

Now we see the third wave of breastfeeding help: the credentialed lactation consultants whose numbers have mushroomed, medical researchers and practitioners who are advancing the field, and the Academy of Breastfeeding Medicine as a formal organization. *The Breastfeeding Mother's Guide to Making More Milk* combines all these resources for mothers who may otherwise never find their way past the hurdles of low self-confidence and inexperienced helpers. As the field of lactation has come into its own as a specialty, more and more of the previously "hopeless" cases have been successfully addressed and remedied, many of them completely, and many mothers, no longer hopeless, are able to achieve a full milk supply for their babies. The ones that don't get a full supply usually experience enough of an improvement to make the effort well worthwhile.

Whatever the circumstances are, or whatever the root problem, you can find your situation in this book and, detective-style and systematically, alone or with support from your health care professionals, make the changes necessary to turn the problem around. This book shows us how almost anyone can make more milk.

—Martha Sears, RN

Acknowledgments

This book was a four-year labor of love and a compilation of the expertise and experience of many colleagues, friends, and clients. A big debt of gratitude is owed to Flossie Rollhauser, Karen Zeretske, and Ann Conlon-Smith, who were the first of several lactation professionals to enthusiastically urge us to write this book because there was no thorough low-milk-production resource for either mothers or health care professionals.

We wish to express our deep appreciation to our amazing agent, Maura Kye-Casella, who saw our vision and knew how much mothers need this book; our brilliant editor, Judith McCarthy, who shared the vision and worked tirelessly to help us craft the book to its greatest potential; and Martha Sears, who wrote such a wonderful foreword and gave us invaluable support and guidance. We are indebted to Jan Barger for her expert review and editorial advice, Teresa Pitman for her talented editorial help in a pinch, Diana Cassar-Uhl and Norma Ritter for their gracious editorial assistance on the early drafts, and Becky Krumwiede, Katy Lebbing, and Victoria Nesterova for their assistance in digging up the research articles that were critical to our understanding and new insights. We owe Taina Litwak our warmest thanks for providing the gorgeous technical illustrations and graciously lending her fabulous cabin on the island of Vinalhaven, Maine, for the writing retreat where our dreams and ideas first took form.

We thank Catherine Watson Genna for generously sharing her insights of the physiology and microanatomy of lactation and dysfunctional suck issues, Diane Wiessinger for her innovative insights into optimal latching and the language of teaching lactation concepts, and Nancy Williams, Cynthia Good-Mojab, and Dr. Kathleen Kendall-Tackett for their fascinating insights from the dual perspective of both lactation and psychotherapy.

In addition to those already mentioned, the following are among the great minds we thank for their contributions to this book: Dr. James Akre, Dr. Pamela Berens, Christine Betzold, Kelly Bonyata, Jan Ellen Brown, Nancy Jo Bykowski, Dr. Elizabeth Coryllos, Jean Cotterman, Suzanne Cox, Dr. Randall Craig, Arnetta Dailey, Victoria Fisher, Dr. Mona Gabbay, Dr. Lawrence Gartner, Dr. Donna Geddes, Lenore Goldfarb, Dr. Marilyn Grams, Karen Gromada, Lynnette Hafken, Dr. Thomas Hale, Dr. Peter Hartmann, Patricia Hatherly, Barbara Heaney, Kathryn Higgins, Teresa Himes, Dr. Elliot Hirsch, Kay Hoover, Judy Hopkinson, Sheila Humphrey, Hilary Jacobson, Dee Kassing, Dr. Jackie Kent, Awtar Kaur Khalsa, Laura Larocca, Samantha Leeson, Chele Marmet, Dr. James McKenna, Julia Mennella, Dr. Leon Mitoulas, Nancy Mohrbacher, Dr. James Murphy, Dr. Frank Nice, Dr. Brian Palmer, Dr. Ann Perrine, Linda Pohl, Cheryl Scott, Ellen Shell, Terriann Shell, Patricia Shelly, Dr. Christina Smillie, Linda Smith, Debra Swank, Solveig Steen, Tamar Sternfeld, Jennifer Tow, Mechell Turner, Julie Wagner, Dr. Corrine Welt, Margaret Wills, Barbara Wilson-Clay, and Lynn Wolf.

Finally, we're grateful to Emily Torgerson, Sylvia Ellison, Rocio Camargo-Ruiz, Diane Herman, Gina Stubbs, Angela Cannon, and all the mothers who shared their stories with us, as well as all our clients and their babies from whom we've learned so much.

Diana's Personal Acknowledgments

I am grateful to my dear online sisterhood, the source of my greatest support, inspiration, and entertainment. I owe my most profound thanks to my cherished sons, Alex, Ben, and Quinn, who enrich my life in countless ways and are sweetly patient while I work on my books, and my dear husband, Brad, who is always supportive of my work to help breastfeeding mothers, who is happy to cook or order takeout when dinner isn't ready because I've been buried in book work again, and whom I love so very much for these and countless other reasons. I would also like to extend a note of deep gratitude to my father, Davis, late mother, Mary, and brother, John, who are the foundation of love that taught me there is no greater accomplishment than serving others.

Lisa's Personal Acknowledgments

I would like to thank all who have contributed to my learning over the years. The Wise Women Lactation Consultants group shared their expertise and acted as a sounding board for ideas new and old, along with the professional liaison department of La Leche League of Southern California/Nevada, who have been by my side from the beginning and shared their wisdom as well as cheered me on as ideas unfolded and the book was born. If it takes a village to raise a child, it takes the support of great mentors and friends to write a book such as this. I am also grateful to the members of the Breastfeeding and Herbs e-mail list for lactation professionals, who came up with hard-to-find research, and the mothers of Mothers Overcoming Breastfeeding Issues (MOBI), who provide real-life feedback on what works for them.

Most of all, I am grateful to my family for putting up with mom "being in the cave" as I researched, wrote, and edited. My dear husband, Tom, cooked many meals and held down the fort while working long hours and going to school, and my remaining children at home, Stephanie and Eric, helped keep house when I wasn't available and came through when I needed them the most. Though not here in body, my older sons, Chris and Ryan, along with Chris's wife, Channyn, all provided frequent moral support.

Introduction

A new baby! What an exciting time in your life! Naturally, you want your baby to have the very best, which is why you've decided to breastfeed. But like many breastfeeding mothers, you may wonder if you can produce enough milk. In fact, concerns about making enough milk are the most common questions on breastfeeding hotlines and the number one reason mothers offer supplement or give up breastfeeding altogether.

For a long time, it was assumed that mothers who worried about their milk production just didn't understand how breastfeeding worked and that all they needed was a little education and reassurance to get breastfeeding back on track. You may have read books or websites that addressed questions about low milk production with this presumption. Maybe someone even told you the problem was really all in your mind.

While it's true that most mothers can make enough milk, we are now learning that there are definitely mothers who really aren't making enough milk, and for a variety of reasons, their numbers may be rising. We're also discovering that there are more causes for low milk production than we once realized. Fortunately, there are also more ways to solve these problems. This book will address all the major concerns about milk supply and help you develop strategies to improve your situation.

Milk Supply Myths, Truths, and Misunderstandings

Like so many other things, our understanding of breastfeeding is influenced by cultural beliefs that have a powerful effect on our feelings and behavior. We have a tendency to accept what society says as true, but the fact is that not everything our culture believes is accurate. Learning to distinguish between breastfeeding myths and truths helps us to understand more clearly what is happening and find the best solution.

Mothers in Western cultures often hear worrisome stories of friends who "didn't have enough milk" or whose milk "dried up," leading them to wonder if it could happen to them. It is also common to hear that if you don't eat a perfect diet or drink the right amount of fluids, then your milk will be inadequate. Our distrust in nature has even led some to believe that modern women have evolved to a point where they're no longer capable of nourishing a baby completely at the breast. But the truth is that evolution doesn't happen in just a few generations.

Mothers sometimes hear that women in their family haven't been able to make enough milk, and they worry that it might be an inheritable trait. Genetics can occasionally play a role, but more often the true cause of milk production failure in the family tree is only a few generations old and based on poor information and mismanagement of breastfeeding rather than family genes.

One of the most problematic myths is that breastfeeding must be "all or nothing": either you must choose to breastfeed exclusively or else you should only feed formula, because doing both is too hard and not worth the effort. This kind of thinking unnecessarily eliminates options that allow babies to receive at least some human milk when exclusive breastfeeding is difficult or impossible. Another common belief is that a mother is stuck with her "equipment," and if her body is struggling to make enough milk, there isn't much she can do to increase her supply. The truth is that there are often ways to improve milk production, and it's certainly worth trying.

Why Some Mothers Can't Make Enough Milk

Humans are mammals, and inadequate milk production is rare among mammals. *So why do so many women seem to have problems making enough milk?* Lactation is clearly a successful part of the human biological design, or we would not have survived as a species. Yet, though we're clearly designed to breastfeed successfully, the fact remains that some women simply do not make enough milk.

The answer may lie in distinguishing between the internal and external causes of low milk production. *Secondary problems* occur when a mother starts with a full milk supply, or at least the capacity to make a full supply of milk, and then something happens to interfere with the process. *Primary problems* originate within the mother's body. Naturally, some overlapping may occur, but most causes fit into these two categories.

Primary causes are often the most puzzling. We now live in a world that is full of pollution, chemicals, pesticides, and medications that are capable of interfering with our hormones, including those that affect breast development and milk production. Technological advances allow us to overcome infertility problems and help women have babies yet overlook whether the breast might be affected as well. And there are other biological reasons that a woman's milk production may be suppressed.

You may feel confident that you already know why you're not making enough milk. If you had breast reduction, for instance, you may assume that your surgery reduced your ability to make milk. But do you have sore nipples? A poor latch could exacerbate an already fragile milk supply situation. What if you also have a thyroid problem, another primary cause? As you read this book, we encourage you to consider all possible causes. Sometimes there are multiple reasons, and your milk production may not be able to be increased effectively unless each cause is identified and addressed.

One of the most helpful concepts introduced in this book is the Milk Supply Equation, a compilation of all the factors that are necessary for adequate milk production. This equation is explained in Chapter 1, and the appropriate sections are highlighted in later chapters as each category of low milk supply causes is discussed to help you narrow down your search. Consider this your "cheat sheet" as you work through the book.

What Can Be Done About Low Milk Production

In the past, mothers were often told that there was little that could be done to help them and that it wasn't worth the effort to breast-feed anyway. However, research has proved that your milk is the very best food for your baby and that some is better than none. It's not necessary to have a full milk supply to have a satisfying breast-feeding experience.

Fortunately, new advances in the field of lactation are helping us to develop better strategies—it is rarely too late. While the concepts presented in this book reflect the most current knowledge, our understanding of lactation is continually changing, and new developments will enable mothers to improve their milk production even more effectively in the future. Where available, we present information that is "evidence-based," meaning there are valid research studies to support the information. However, we also present remedies for increasing milk production that have long been considered effective by traditional societies but have not been validated scientifically so that you can evaluate all potential options for increasing your milk production. It will be up to you and your health care advisers to determine what is appropriate for your circumstances.

A critical concept introduced in this book is the importance of targeting your treatment strategy to the cause of your low supply. Without understanding why you aren't able to produce enough milk, you may easily put time, effort, and money into solutions that don't address the real problem. When your strategy doesn't work, you might then incorrectly conclude that your low milk production is irreversible. Strategic targeting will increase your chances for success.

Your Navigators Toward Higher Milk Production

The experience of not having enough milk and the journey toward finding solutions can feel very lonely, but as you read this book, you'll be in the company of two women who understand your situation well. Our passion for this topic comes from our firsthand experience. Diana West had breast reduction surgery and was unable to produce enough milk for her first son, Alex, but did have enough milk for her second and third babies, Ben and Quinn. Lisa Marasco, on the other hand, had three uneventful breastfeeding experiences with Christopher, Ryan, and Stephanie before experiencing a mysterious drop in milk supply during the second half year of Eric's life.

Along with our personal knowledge of low milk production, we bring our professional knowledge and expertise as International Board Certified Lactation Consultants (IBCLC) to help you navigate the path toward making more milk. We don't presume to have all the answers and cures for every low-milk-production problem. Some cases are very complex, and, as with removing the layers on an onion, it can take a lot of peeling to find the core problem. You also may hit dead ends before getting to the root cause and have to go back a step or two and reconsider ideas you had discarded. A lot of persistence and detective work are sometimes required. We understand, though, that sometimes our best efforts are not enough, nor are all mothers emotionally or realistically able to take all the steps necessary to reach their breastfeeding goals.

Throughout this journey, keep in mind that you are an important member of your own health care team. You may discover concepts and strategies that others have not had an opportunity to explore. At the same time, do consult with experts, as they may have additional information. Access all the resources that are available to you, because they may hold pieces to the puzzle that this book cannot provide.

An important theme in this book is the tremendous value of your milk. By deciding to breastfeed, you have made a commitment to giving your baby the best of yourself. Every drop of your milk is a gift with lifetime benefits. We cannot promise every mother a full milk supply, but the concepts we share here will help you find greater satisfaction with your breastfeeding relationship. Most of all, remember that success lies not with ounces but with love. What a lucky baby you have whose mother is making the effort to give him the best of herself!

We've referred to all babies in this book as "he" only to make it easier to tell whom we are referring to because all mothers are obviously "she." If your baby is a girl, please kiss her for us and tell her that no matter how many times we say "he" in this book, we adore baby girls just as much as baby boys.

We want to hear your story! Please visit our website, www.lowmilksupply .org, to share your feedback about what has and has not worked for your particular breastfeeding situation. With your help, we will have more answers for future mothers and babies.

Investigating Your Milk Supply

Sylvia's Story

With my first baby, Windom, I had preeclampsia and ended up in the ICU, so we were separated for most of the first twenty-four hours. He was sleepy and not very interested in feeding. The ICU nurse said not to pump because I wouldn't produce much milk at first anyway.

When we were discharged, the pediatrician told me the expected weight gain was 1 to 3 ounces (30 to 90 milliliters) per *day*! This seems laughable now, but I didn't know better then, so I really thought something might be wrong with my milk because he wasn't gaining 3 ounces a day. My mom believed that my milk wasn't rich enough because she had been told this about her milk when I was a baby. The pediatricians kept bringing us back every two days for weight checks and said I should nurse Windom every three hours, followed by .5 to 1 ounce (15 to 30 milliliters) of formula. When I mentioned my nipple soreness, I was told the best treatment was to limit his time at the breast.

My incredibly supportive sister urged me to get help, so when Windom was one week old, we saw a lactation consultant. After a few weeks of improved latch and more frequent feedings, Windom was doing fine, meeting all developmental milestones, and gaining weight at the lower but acceptable end of normal range.

Things were very different with my second baby, Harper, who seemed to want to nurse every time I blinked my eyes for the first six weeks. After going through the sleepy baby stuff with Windom, I was glad to have a baby who was ready to nurse, nurse, nurse. I knew I would not revisit any doubts about supply.

CHAPTER 1

Understanding Your Milk Factory

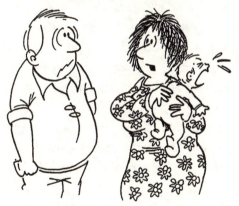

THE MORE HE CRIES THE LESS MILK HE DRINKS,
SO THE LESS MILK IS PRODUCED,
SO THERE'S LESS FOR HIM TO DRINK,
SO HE CRIES BECAUSE HE DIDN'T GET A DRINK.
DO YOU UNDERSTAND THAT?

Just like the father in this cartoon, many of us feel confused and perplexed when it comes to understanding our breasts and our babies and whether everything is OK or not. But knowledge is power! When you understand how your body builds and runs your milk factory, you'll have a head start on solving your own personal puzzle. Even if you already know a lot, chances are you'll find even deeper insights in this up-to-date, research-based information about milk production.

Seasons of Breast Development: Growing a Milk Factory

Human milk production—your milk factory—is an amazing process that is built upon the foundation of mammary gland (breast) development that began before you were born. While most mammals have fully developed mammary glands prior to pregnancy, the human breast develops in stages and does not reach full operational maturity until pregnancy. Somewhat like a fruit tree in winter with only a few leaves and dormant buds, the nonlactating breast has large and small branches called *ducts* and *ductules*, along with a small number of leaves, the *alveoli*, that contain the milk-making cells. Each of the several main branches, the ducts, together with its smaller branches, the ductules, and leaves, the alveoli, form *lobes* that intertwine yet function somewhat independently of each other.

During pregnancy, the color of the areola and nipple deepen, and the areola often enlarges in size. Small bumps called Montgomery glands, which may circle or dot the areola and are often unnoticeable until pregnancy, also grow in size. The veins along the surface of the breast become more prominent, appearing both larger and bluer. Internally, alveoli multiply and grow, filling out the lobes inside the breast like a tree leafing out in springtime. You may notice your breasts growing larger or becoming firmer as this happens. Breast tenderness is common and a positive sign that all is working normally. If growth occurs quickly and is substantial, reddish or purplish stretch marks may develop that later fade over time.

When baby is born, milk production kicks into high gear, and the tree bears its crop of fruit, the milk. The milk-making cells may continue to multiply according to the demand for milk during the next several weeks, causing additional breast growth. As baby grows older and his need gradually diminishes, the milk-making parts of the tree begin to slow down and recede. This is the autumn season of the breast, when there is still milk-making activity, but at a lower level. At weaning, the breast gradually returns to its resting winter state, awaiting a new season of pregnancy.

The driving forces underlying this cycle are hormones. From puberty on, the waxing and waning of *estrogen* and *progesterone* during your menstrual cycle slowly, over time, develop the ducts and alveoli further. This subtle stimulation continues until about age thirty-five. Pregnancy causes a much larger rise in both of these hormones, as well as the production of *prolactin, human placental lactogen* (hPL), *human chorionic gonadotropin* (hCG), and *growth hormone*, which all help to stimulate glandular growth. Changes in breast size during pregnancy are most closely related to the concentration of human placental lactogen, which is produced only by the placenta and so only during pregnancy. This makes your placenta a crucial player in the construction of a good milk factory for baby. Other key hormones that play a role in stimulating mammary development include *insulin, cortisol,* and *thyroid hormones.*

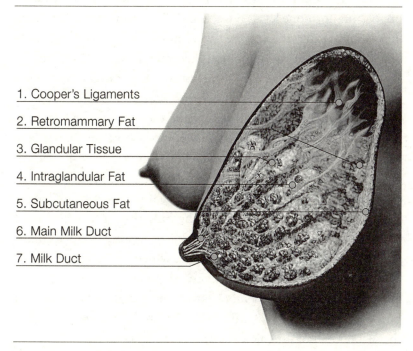

1. Cooper's Ligaments

2. Retromammary Fat

3. Glandular Tissue

4. Intraglandular Fat

5. Subcutaneous Fat

6. Main Milk Duct

7. Milk Duct

Anatomy of the lactating breast

Hormones and the Milk-Making Process

Understanding how your hormones function helps you know if they are helping or hindering your milk supply. Each hormone has one or more types of corresponding receptors located wherever its influence is needed. The two must bind together like keys that fit only into locks that are configured for them. There must also be a good match between the amount of hormone and the number of receptors; a lot of keys and few locks are not effective, and a few keys but a lot of locks are not effective. The number of available receptors can change and is influenced by various factors. In addition, the ease in which hormones and receptors bind together can also vary; a well-oiled lock turns easily, but a rusty one does not. Type 2 diabetes is one example of a rusty lock problem that occurs when insulin receptors resist binding to insulin; we call this *insulin resistance*. Pregnancy and lactation cause many changes in the number and binding ability of hormone receptors important to breast development and milk production. Because receptors are equally important, hormone levels provide only half the picture. Yet, since hormones are easy to measure with simple blood tests, this is usually all we look at to judge how well our hormonal systems are functioning. It's not as easy to measure the number of receptors because this would require taking an actual tissue sample.

Many hormones are involved in *lactogenesis*, the process of making milk. Like ingredients in a cake recipe, some hormones play minor roles while others are crucial for a good result. Prolactin, the major milk-stimulating hormone, is normally present in small amounts in our bodies, but its level gradually rises quite high during pregnancy, peaking at birth. The only reason that the breast doesn't make lots of milk at this point is because the placenta is producing high levels of progesterone, which interferes with prolactin's receptors on the milk-making cells and prevents the prolactin "keys" from having much effect. Instead, *colostrum*, your first milk, is produced. This earliest phase of milk production during the second half of pregnancy is known as *lactogenesis I*.

Since the placenta makes the majority of the progesterone during pregnancy, progesterone drops quickly once the placenta comes out, allowing prolactin to start doing its work. Within thirty to forty hours, the change to full milk production begins, and mothers usually notice an increase in milk volume between the second and fourth day. This milk is lighter in color, thinner, and more watery than colostrum. When this happens, *lactogenesis II* has begun, and women say that their milk has "come in." Full milk production requires prolactin, insulin, and cortisol.

This gradual increase in milk production is a perfect match for your baby's slowly expanding stomach. During his first day of life, he may take as little as one-half teaspoon (2.5 milliliters) or as much as 4 ounces (120 milliliters) of colostrum. After the second day, intake usually increases rapidly to between 13 and 29 ounces (384 and 858 milliliters) by the end of the first week, eventually settling to an average of 25 to 27 ounces (750 to 800 milliliters) per day.[1] This amount stays about the same from the end of the first month until baby begins solids and needs less milk. Even though he may take more some days than others, especially during growth spurts, he doesn't need increasing amounts of milk overall because his rate of growth slows down 50 percent by four to six months, making the amount he takes at one month enough for when he is older as well.

Milk Ejection: Nature's Delivery System

Every time baby suckles, nerves in the nipple and areola send messages to the brain that trigger the pituitary to release *oxytocin*. This hormone causes muscle-like cells around the alveoli to contract and squeeze milk down the ducts for delivery to the baby. This process of releasing milk is called *milk ejection*, often referred to as *let-down*. Without this reflex, little milk can be removed, and when not removed well, the breast receives the message to cut back on milk production. Milk ejection is a critical component of the big picture of milk production and works extremely well the vast majority of time. The few situations that can negatively affect milk ejection and lead to lower milk production are explored in Chapter 10.

Milk ejections are not onetime events but rather can be triggered multiple times during a breastfeeding or pumping session. Babies generally learn to anticipate whatever pattern their mothers' milk ejections follow. A hungry baby will continue to suckle off and on when the milk is not flowing strongly, hoping to trigger another ejection. In the early days, however, some babies may become upset if the milk ejection reflex does not happen quickly, pulling away in anger or frustration. Over time and with positive experiences, baby learns to trust the breast, while his mother learns to trust that her milk will flow. Both begin to relax into a confident breastfeeding relationship. When milk production and flow are low, some babies may remain distrustful until the flow is improved, compounding the difficulty in getting breastfeeding going.

Oxytocin release that stimulates milk ejection is unique in that it is not controlled exclusively by sensory (touch) stimulation but can also be triggered by thoughts and feelings. Many breastfeeding mothers can attest to this when a crying baby in a shopping center triggers a let-down and they notice wet spots on their shirts!

One other interesting aspect is how milk ejections affect the appearance of your milk. You've probably heard about *foremilk*, the low-fat "skim milk," and *hindmilk*, the high-fat, creamier milk at the end of a feeding. These terms make it sound as if the breast produces two kinds of milk, but that's not the case. As milk is made, the fat globules stick to the sides of the alveoli where the milk is stored and are flushed out gradually with milk ejections. The milk your baby receives in the beginning has less fat and a higher percentage of lactose, an important milk sugar, but the longer he feeds on a breast, the more cream he receives, ending up with a nicely balanced meal.

How Your Body Decides How Much Milk to Make

So how do the breasts figure out how much milk to make? Some mothers seem to initially make enough for two babies, while others start off with a lower volume that gradually increases to meet baby's needs. At the same time that baby's suckling triggers the release of oxytocin for milk ejection, the pituitary gland also releases a surge of prolactin to encourage continued resupplying of the breast. This is necessary because the body is constantly clearing out hormones from our system. In the weeks following birth, prolactin decreases until it reaches a lower plateau, but the more often prolactin surges, the higher the average circulating level, or *baseline prolactin*, will be. At the same time, receptors for prolactin multiply. The development of prolactin receptors in the breast is believed to be related to the frequency of early suckling stimulation and milk removal: the more often baby breastfeeds in the first days and weeks after birth, the more receptors are made.[2] Good receptor development is critical to sustaining long-term milk production.

When prolactin is dropping and its receptors are being established, the milk-making process changes from being largely hormone driven (*endocrine*) to more locally controlled in the breast (*autocrine*), responding to baby's demand by adjusting the rate of milk production up or down according to how much and how often milk is taken out. The goal of the autocrine process is to fine-tune, or *calibrate*, milk production to meet baby's actual needs, with a little to spare. Lactation consultant Catherine Watson Genna, B.S., IBCLC, explains that like the marketing research department for a factory, your body spends the first few weeks after baby is born determining whether it needs more or fewer assembly lines to meet baby's milk needs. In essence, all the early experiences of how often baby nurses and how much milk he removes is part of the body's "market research phase" for calibrating your milk production. *The more milk that you remove during this time, the higher your milk supply will be calibrated.* This is critical in developing the final blueprint for a milk-making factory that will ultimately meet baby's needs.

Baby Calls the Shots

The breast works by a process of demand and supply: baby suckles when he wants milk, the breast delivers it via milk ejection, and then more milk is made to replace what was taken. If baby has taken all the milk and keeps asking for more, additional milk will be made. Calibration is the body's process of figuring out how much milk to make and is designed to be an *infant-driven* system. This is why women may have very different breastfeeding and milk production experiences from one baby to the next. Each baby provides a new set of cues that triggers production, setting into motion a new and unique experience. Similarly, the larger-producing side can change from one baby to the next. Interestingly, mothers of baby boys tend to produce more milk than mothers of baby girls due to the fact that boys seem to grow a little faster and need a little more, thus creating a bigger milk supply in their mothers.[3] The ability of a woman's body to respond to baby's milk-making signals depends not only on baby having free access to the breast to send the signals but also on mother's body having well-functioning nerves to carry the signals from the breast to the brain for processing. It is truly an amazing, coordinated dance between a mother and her infant.

The Resource-Efficient Breast

Your body does not like to waste precious resources. It works very hard to find a good balance of milk production that is enough for baby, plus a safety cushion, by sensitively monitoring the degree of fullness of the breast. The "golden rule of milk production" is that *the emptier the breast is kept, the harder the body works to restock and the higher the rate of production.* If a factory's warehouse keeps emptying and orders are pouring in, management will hire new workers and speed up the production lines. Your breast tissue may actually grow, adding new machinery.[4] Of course, these adjustments require a little time when baby is asking for more milk than is available. On the other hand, if the breast's warehouse is consistently overflowing, management may begin to downsize the factory by reducing the number of assembly lines and laying off workers.

This happens because concentrations of a whey protein called the *feedback inhibitor of lactation* (FIL) increase as the breast fills up.

The more FIL rises, the slower the breast makes milk, much like we slow the water down in a bathtub that is filling up too quickly. Concentrations of FIL are low when the breast is empty, telling the breast to produce milk faster, just as we turn the water faucet on high when the bathtub is empty and we want to fill it up.

If demand appears to have dropped permanently due to little or no nursing or pumping, management may even close the factory completely. We call this process of the breast permanently getting rid of some or all of the workers and equipment *involution*. For a period of time, this downward trend of milk production may be reversible, but after a while it is not, depending on individual factors. This is why a breast that becomes engorged needs to have milk removed on a regular basis; it is possible to go from too much to very little or no milk in a short time. This is also why it isn't a good idea to "wait until the breast fills up" before feeding baby. More milk might build up initially, but ultimately milk production will slow down, and less will be made in the end.

Even when the baby seems to have removed all available milk from the breast, if he continues to suckle, he will get whatever milk is being made and released at the moment. It's as if the bathtub drain is open but the spigot is on. However, milk flow is greatly reduced when there is little accumulated milk in the breast. Even though the rate of milk production is high, thirsty babies often become impatient and fussy when the milk flow is slower. Mothers frequently misinterpret this scenario and conclude that their breasts are empty and not giving milk. More likely, there is a constant production of milk—it's just that the milk is being delivered slower than baby desires.

The Role of Storage Capacity

The maximum amount of milk that can be stored before the breast says "stop!" is your *storage capacity* and is determined by the amount of fully developed glands inside the breast rather than exterior breast size.[5] Storage capacity, the warehouse for the milk factory, can change and may increase during the first few months depend-

Why Does One Side Produce More than the Other?

One of the most common observations of nursing mothers is that one breast makes more milk than the other. In fact, it is rare for two breasts to produce exactly the same amount of milk. More often, one side, usually the right, makes significantly more milk than the other. While baby can certainly create a larger supply on one side by his preference, this happens even in women whose breasts are equally stimulated by exclusive pumping. If it bothers you, try to alternate starting breasts so that both receive equal stimulation. Or, you can even try starting on the lower producer every time to even production out. But don't be surprised if one continues to be a "superproducer." It's perfectly normal.

ing on baby's appetite. Storage capacity is also one of the biggest factors in determining how often babies need to feed. Babies of mothers who have smaller warehouses need to feed more often, while babies of mothers with large-capacity warehouses have the option of eating larger meals less often.

Does Milk Production Have an Upper Limit?

Unfortunately, we don't have the complete answer on upper limits of human milk production because researchers have not yet explored this subject matter. In theory, according to the demand-and-supply principle of lactation, the more milk that is removed, the more milk should be made. However, ultimately there are limiting constraints. Some women's capabilities are limited because their bodies didn't develop a lot of basic glandular tissue during puberty. Some started with enough, but for some reason that tissue didn't blossom well in response to pregnancy hormones. Others simply don't have enough functional ducts and nerves because of previous breast surgery. Still, why doesn't the functional tissue that exists just produce higher and higher levels of milk when prompted to do so? Part of the answer may lie in the fact that milk supply is calibrated according to the amount and frequency of milk removal during the early weeks, within the limitations of overall breast tissue. Some women seem to have great flexibility and can easily increase milk production with additional stimulation for quite a while after delivery, while other women seem to have a short window of calibration, so that their milk production reaches a plateau and is not as responsive to demands for more milk. Apparently, these women's breasts begin losing some of their "leaves" earlier than others do.[6]

The Milk Supply Equation

The components necessary for good milk production can be summed up in this equation:

The Milk Supply Equation

Sufficient glandular tissue
+ Intact nerve pathways *and* ducts
+ Adequate hormones *and* hormone receptors
+ Adequately frequent, effective milk removal and stimulation

= GOOD MILK PRODUCTION

If one part of this equation isn't there, milk production can be compromised. If more than one part falters, the possibility of problems is greater. Sometimes boosting another area of the equation can compensate for an area that is missing or low, though not always, because each one of these factors is necessary for good milk production.

Milk Production Is Designed to Succeed

We hope you now have a good understanding of how your breasts make milk and how you and your baby influence the process of milk production. As you read through the next chapters, keep in mind that nature designed lactation to be a robust process with multiple safety nets. If one part of the milk-making factory isn't functioning optimally, another will work harder to compensate. This is why most mothers around the world breastfeed very successfully even under circumstances that are less than ideal. It is only when there are numerous breakdowns in the system or one problem is particularly severe that mothers and babies have difficulty breastfeeding. In most cases, keeping mother and baby together whenever possible so that they can respond to each other's cues will be key in getting things back on track. But if you are feeling confused about your baby's behavior or what's happening with your breasts, the next chapter will help you determine what's normal and what's not.

CHAPTER 2

What's Normal and What's Not

What's "normal" for breastfeeding and what isn't seems to be a common source of confusion. Sometimes mothers think they aren't making enough milk when they really are because they misinterpret their babies' behaviors. By the time we hear everyone else's opinion on what should be considered normal, it's hard to know who or what to believe.

For better or worse, our first teachers for how to interpret baby behavior are our own mothers, family, and friends. Unless you have a medical background or formal training in child development, you'll probably rely on their advice as you assess your own baby's behavior for the first time. This can be helpful, but it can also be frustrating because their ideas may be out of date or they may have conflicting opinions. Grandma tells you that the baby is crying after feeding because he ate too much and his stomach is upset. Your neighbor tells you that the baby didn't get enough to eat and is still hungry. Your best friend warns you that the baby may be allergic to your milk. Aunt Susie thinks the baby is "colicky" and just needs to "cry it out." Which interpretation is true? Which are you more likely to believe if you're already worried about making enough milk?

Normal Baby Behaviors After the Milk Comes In

☐ Baby breastfeeds at least eight to twelve times in twenty-four hours, spaced approximately two to three hours apart, but sometimes clustered together.

☐ Baby sleeps no more than one four- to five-hour stretch once a day until breastfeeding is well established and he is growing appropriately.

☐ Baby begins feedings with a few quick suckles, followed by bursts of several sucks with long, drawing jaw movements that pause momentarily so baby can swallow.

☐ Baby's swallows can be heard frequently as a whispered "kuh" or a gulping sound in the first five to ten minutes, then less frequently thereafter.

☐ Baby breastfeeds actively for approximately fifteen to forty minutes per feeding but sometimes less if milk flow is very fast.

☐ Baby seems to drain one breast thoroughly before taking the other side, or he may not take the second breast at all.

The only true way to know if baby is getting enough is by evaluating his weight gain and diaper output. Baby's behaviors do also provide clues, but when you have a good understanding of normal baby and breastfeeding behaviors, misinterpretations and misperceptions are less likely to happen. This chapter will help you sort through the realities and myths of normal breastfeeding.

Commonly Misinterpreted Baby Behaviors

There are many common infant behaviors that can mislead you to believe that your baby isn't getting enough milk if you don't understand what baby may really be saying.

Frequent Feedings

It's normal for babies to breastfeed frequently, especially during the early weeks. In the first two days, baby may nurse as often as every half hour, *counting from the beginning of one feeding to the beginning of the next*. The actual feeding is usually for only short periods, with baby waking to feed at night more than during the day. After the milk comes in, most babies begin feeding every two to three hours, or eight to twelve times in twenty-four hours, on average, though some cultures expect and allow a baby to breastfeed as often as several times in an hour. Newborns aren't as efficient as they will be later on, and they also need to gain weight faster than they ever will again. How often would you need to eat if you were trying to double your weight in six months and triple it in a year? Babies need frequent opportunities to feed in order to fuel all that growth.

Parents often expect babies to feed at regular intervals around the clock, but some babies will nurse several times over a period of a few hours and then take an extra long nap. These *cluster feeds* can occur at any time but happen most often in the late afternoon and evening. Of course, never being satisfied and always wanting to be at the breast *can* indicate that baby isn't getting enough. You'll know if frequent nursing is a problem or not by looking at diaper output and weight gain, as explained in the next chapter.

Frequency Days and Growth Spurts

Many babies will have "frequency days" when they seem extra fussy and want to nurse much more frequently than their usual pattern. You may even feel like you're "running out of milk" because your breasts are soft, when it's actually the reverse: your breasts feel soft because baby is feeding so often that he is not allowing much milk to accumulate. The positive side of this is that he is stimulating a higher rate of milk production.

Remember your teenage days? Mom would buy a certain amount of groceries each week. Then, suddenly, you started eating ravenously, and before the week was up, the cupboards were bare, and you were searching for more food. Were you starving to death? No, you were just extra hungry, and the stockpile of groceries was temporarily depleted. All that was needed was an extra trip to the grocery store to meet your additional needs. When the growth spurt stopped, your appetite returned to normal. It's the same with babies.

Frequency days generally happen around two to three weeks, six weeks, three months, and six months, with baby usually returning to his previous feeding pattern in three to seven days. It was once thought that these spurts were baby's way of increasing milk production to meet his growing needs, much like bottle-fed babies tend to take more formula over time. However, we now know that babies stimulate temporary increases in milk production that settle back down again when the growth spurt is over.[1]

Less Frequent Feedings

While frequent feedings worry some mothers, others become concerned that they must not have enough milk when their baby begins to nurse less frequently. If a newborn is feeding fewer than eight times a day after the first few days of life, it *is* possible that he is conserving calories because he isn't getting enough milk. But more often, a growing baby is able to take larger feedings, allowing him to go longer between meals. This may be especially true if you have a large storage capacity, allowing baby to take as much as he can handle in a single feeding. Diaper output will usually tell you which is the case.

Short Feedings

Perhaps you've heard that baby must feed for a specific amount of time at each breast in order to get enough milk or to get to the "hindmilk." This isn't true, because all babies and breasts respond differently. Some babies are able to transfer large amounts of milk in as little as five to ten minutes, particularly when the mother has a strong milk flow. After the first few weeks, shorter feedings may also be a matter of baby simply having learned how to nurse more efficiently so that he gets the same amount of milk in less time. Or he may be "snacking" in between longer feedings or as part of a cluster feed. Fluctuations in milk supply throughout the day can also affect the length of breastfeeding.

On the other hand, some newborns stop feeding early out of discouragement or fatigue. They may not be able to get milk out easily due to a latching or suck problem, or because the milk isn't flowing as fast as they want or expect after having experienced faster flow from a bottle. Babies can also become frustrated by slow milk flow because the mother's milk production has decreased for some reason.

Baby Cries and Takes a Bottle After Breastfeeding

While an underfed baby may indeed gulp down a bottle after breastfeeding, some will take a bottle even after consuming enough milk at the breast. Is the bottle offered because baby truly needs it or because someone else wants to feed him or *thinks* he needs it? Was baby doing just fine before, and now his having accepted the bottle after a feeding shakes your confidence? Or was he crying, and the bottle seemed to calm him down?

Sometimes what's really happening is that baby is being stuffed into a stupor in a very unnatural way. Just because a bottle stops the fussing doesn't automatically mean that he needs more to eat. Think about how mothers handled this before bottles and formula were invented. Crying can mean things other than hunger; baby may just need more sucking time, or he may have become upset during or after a feeding because of allergies, gas, or reflux. Don't be afraid to call your pediatrician if his crying is worrisome, and be persistent if your gut says that something is wrong and you aren't satisfied with the answers. It isn't always about your milk supply!

Baby Chokes, Sputters, and Arches at the Breast

If your baby chokes and sputters while breastfeeding—perhaps arching and pulling off, crying, or not nursing for long periods at the breast—it could be an indication of *too* much milk! If so, your baby may gain weight rapidly, or his weight gain may be slower due to his struggles with the strong milk flow. He may cry a lot and act very irritable or restless, especially after feeds. Gulping, choking, sputtering, or coughing during breastfeeding are common, as are biting, clamping down, pulling on the nipple, arching, stiffness, or even screaming. Feedings often seem like battles, with baby having a "love-hate" relationship with the breast and nursing fitfully on and off, feeding for only five or ten minutes total. He may burp a lot, spit up after feedings, and be very gassy, and his stools are often green, watery, foamy, or explosive. Your milk may spray forcefully when he comes off the breast, especially early in the feeding. You may feel very full much of the time, even while offering both breasts, and battle plugged ducts that could lead to breast infections. If this sounds familiar, try feeding on one side per feeding for twenty-four hours as a starting point to see if it helps and visit our website, www.lowmilksupply.org, for more information.

Regular Fussiness in the Late Afternoon or Early Evening

In the first three months of life, many breastfed babies fuss in the late afternoon and early evening. Mothers often worry that this is a sign that baby isn't getting enough to eat, especially if their breasts feel deflated. As discussed in Chapter 1, the most likely explanation for this common phenomenon is that your milk reserves have been drained throughout the day and baby is now withdrawing milk as it is actively made. In fact, this is more likely to happen if you have a larger storage capacity and baby sleeps longer at night and then removes milk faster than it is being made during the daytime in order to get all his meals in.[2]

When there is little accumulated milk in the breasts, the force of the milk flow is reduced. Think of how a water balloon expels water forcibly when full but more slowly when there is less water in it. Since babies often prefer a faster flow of milk when they are hungry, they may become impatient and irritable when the flow is slower late in the day. This fussy time may also coincide with tiredness and overstimulation, which decrease their patience and contribute to crankiness. When offered a bottle at this time, baby may take it eagerly, reinforcing fears that he's starving. Most of the time, the reality is that you have plenty of milk over twenty-four hours, just not a lot right now, *and that's OK.*

Early evening "fussiness" can also be the result of a frustrated infant whose mother is refusing to offer the breast again because baby "just fed." Nursing frequently may be baby's way of compensating for less available milk at the end of the day; if large meals are not available, lots of smaller ones will do. Frequent feeding also may be his way of tanking up before a long sleep. If he calms down right away when put to the breast, the problem more likely is about unrealistic expectations.

To get the most milk possible into baby during this time, try breast compressions to increase the force of the flow (see Chapter 5) and then alternate with cuddles, movement, and singing. Sooner or later, baby will fall into a long, deep sleep. You can also try a galactogogue (milk-stimulating) herbal tea (see Chapter 12) in the late afternoon.

Baby Not Sleeping Through the Night

"Is your baby sleeping through the night?" is one of the first questions new parents hear from friends, relatives, and even from physicians. It stems from a common cultural belief that babies should be sleeping several hours at night as early as three months of age and has become an expectation and measurement of parenting success. Some people even define a "good baby" as one who sleeps through the night. However, sleeping for longer than four hours more than once or twice per twenty-four hours in the first month may indicate baby is not getting enough milk and sleeps to conserve calories.

It is normal for a baby, especially one who is breastfed, to continue to awaken periodically at night during his first year of life. He may nurse one to three times between 10:00 P.M. and 4:00 A.M. and take more milk at night than in the daytime.[3] An important factor in determining how long he can go between feedings is

21

your milk storage capacity and whether you can deliver more milk at a given feeding. Infants of mothers with a large capacity breastfeed less often overall and eventually take a longer break than do infants of mothers with smaller storage capacity.[4]

Many parents report that their baby initially started to sleep longer hours at night only to have that end after a month or two, leaving them to wonder what went wrong. Actually, it really is what "went normal." Remember, there is more going on in baby's life than just eating. The discomfort of teething or an illness can awaken him, searching for comfort. The excitement of increased mobility as he masters rolling over, crawling, or standing can cause him to wake up, looking for mom. Life may just be too exciting in the daytime to eat, so he nurses more at night when the world is dark and less stimulating. If you recently went back to work, baby may also wake more often to make up for missed daytime feedings or even just to touch base and make sure you're still there for him.

Occasionally a change in baby's sleep pattern can indicate that baby needs more food, but there will be other clues to validate this. If nothing has changed in your life, such as starting on a new medication or routine separation from baby, and he is still gaining well and producing lots of diapers, then his sleep pattern is probably related to something other than your milk production.

Reading Baby's Body Language to Gauge Milk Intake

Contentment after a feeding can be a good sign. However, babies who aren't getting enough to eat can sometimes fall asleep and initially *appear* content when they have not taken in enough. How do you tell the difference between a baby who is truly full and one who is apparently content but still hungry? Babies may not speak with their mouths, but they sure do speak through their expressions and posture!

A baby who is getting only a little milk out of the breast will quickly slow down to a "flutter" suck and doze off without letting go of the nipple. He often has a puzzled or worried expression, with furrowed eyebrows and wrinkles in the forehead as if to say,

"Something isn't right; why isn't this working?" as he keeps trying to get more milk. His body never fully relaxes while nursing, and his hands may be tightly fisted and close to his face. If he has difficulty latching on to the breast, he may flail his arms about desperately, adding more chaos to the situation. And when taken off the breast, he may immediately awaken or go through a series of "cluster feeds" that never seem to end. A baby looking for more milk may tug and pull at the breast, or push and knead it with his hands like a kitten. This instinctive behavior is designed to induce another milk ejection, which usually happens if milk is still available. As baby alternately pulls and pushes, he may act "antsy" and unsettled until milk flows again. Less patient (or fed up) babies will come off the breast or even refuse to latch after a while, arching stiffly and screaming as if to say, "Not again! I *told* you this isn't working!" Mothers often interpret this to mean that baby dislikes breastfeeding, but that's not the case at all. Babies are biologically designed to want to breastfeed. What may be frustrating them is not being able to figure out how to get more milk faster.

Another nonverbal message is tightly closed lips, which seem to say, "I'm done for now, thank you." Babies do have their individual limits in how long they are willing to keep trying, and babies born early especially have less stamina. It is important to interpret the messages correctly so that you can change, or help baby to change, what is not working for him right now. When feedings are stressful or filled with conflict, breastfeeding can become a trust issue for the baby. Respecting what he is communicating to you will help rebuild his trust in the breast.

There are also positive baby cues that signal when things are going well for baby. As the milk begins to flow and baby starts swallowing, his eyes open, and the wrinkles and perplexed expression he may have had begin to fade away, as if he is thinking, "Well look at this! I can't believe I'm getting this much! Can it be true?" And as he begins to fill up, baby's fists open up, his arms relax, dropping away from his face, and his eyes slowly close. Mothers often comment on their babies' "milk drunk" expression at the end.

Normal Maternal Breastfeeding Experiences

- ☐ Your breasts felt tender at some point during pregnancy, particularly during the first trimester.
- ☐ Your breasts increased in size.
- ☐ Your areolas darkened.
- ☐ The veins on your breasts became more visible.
- ☐ Your breasts felt fuller, firmer, and perhaps warmer as your milk "came in" between the second and fourth day postpartum.
- ☐ You experienced uterine cramping or gushes of blood, called *lochia*, during feedings in the first few days after birth in response to baby suckling or pumping (these become stronger after each birth).
- ☐ Your breasts feel softer after feedings.

Commonly Misinterpreted Maternal Indicators

Some experiences may lead you to believe that you don't have enough milk, yet they are *not* necessarily reliable signs when taken alone, though several together may indeed be reason to investigate further.

Inability to Pump or Express Much Milk

The amount of milk you can pump may or may not be an accurate measurement of your milk production. Effective pumping depends on the quality of the breast pump, the fit of the kit, the density of the breast tissue, and your overall comfort with and response to pumping. Some mothers release milk very easily to even a low-quality pump and are able to drain their breasts quite well, but most respond best to a consumer- or hospital-grade pump. A few women don't seem to be able to extract milk efficiently with any kind of pump. Pumping can provide some clues to how much milk you are making, but it should not be your only measuring stick. If you are pumping after breastfeeding, baby may have taken most of the available milk. If you've been using a consumer-grade pump and experienced a gradual decrease in milk yield over several weeks or months, it's possible that it may not be your body that is to blame, but rather the pump (see Chapter 11).

Hand expressing to see how much milk you have is also not always an accurate measurement of your milk supply. Hand expression is a skill that can be valuable in stimulating your milk production, but most mothers need practice to become adept at it, and it is still not as effective as a baby who is nursing well.

Little or No Engorgement

A mother who has been nursing frequently from the start does not always feel significant discomfort as her milk comes in, though most mothers do experience some feelings of fullness and warmth. Although you may expect the experience of the milk coming in to be painful, frequent removal of milk often helps to avoid or minimize engorgement.

Not Feeling Milk Ejection

Not all mothers feel the milk ejection reflex happen. When they do, they're more likely to feel those in the beginning as a full breast releases; the sensation tends to dampen with less milk. Leaking from the opposite breast during a feed usually indicates that milk ejection is occurring, especially when the baby begins swallowing audibly at the same time. After several months, sensations of milk ejection often diminish even for those mothers who felt them easily early on.

Not Leaking

Leaking between feedings is not by itself an accurate way to gauge your milk supply. It has more to do with the tension of the muscles in your nipples, which differs from woman to woman, than with milk production. While leaking can be a very positive sign that there is milk in your breasts and some mothers leak more as their milk production increases, leaking alone does not indicate how much milk you have.

Softer Breasts

In the beginning, your breasts may often feel very full before each feeding. After about six weeks, though, the milk supply becomes more harmonious with baby's needs, and the breasts begin to feel softer and less full more of the time (unless it has been an unusually long time between feedings). If you breastfed previously, you may also find that with each new baby your breasts seem to get softer sooner and make this adjustment more quickly.

Milk Wrong Color or Too Thin

Human milk is often somewhat bluish but can vary in color depending on the foods you eat. These variations do not affect the quality of the milk and are certainly not harmful to baby. Fluctuations in the amount of fat in your milk depend on the degree of fullness of the breasts, the time of day, and the age of your baby. Factors such as smoking can also influence the fat content of the milk. However, breastfed babies compensate for these changes by regulating the amount of milk they take. If you have milk that is lower in fat overall, baby will take a larger volume in order to

Where Did My Milk Go?

Baby just came off the breast and needed a little break, but now he's ready for more. You can feel that your breast has milk, but he's fussing, and it isn't flowing. What happened? Without any forces continuing to push or pull the milk out, milk will draw back up into the ducts and ductules like a sponge soaking up water. This can be confusing to both you and baby when the milk is not coming out as it was doing just a little while before. But be reassured that if there was milk there a few minutes ago, it is still there. It just needs a little stimulation for another milk ejection to get things going again.

get enough calories for his needs—assuming he has unrestricted opportunities to nurse.[5]

Do You Have Enough Milk?

Now that you have a good understanding of normal breastfeeding, the next chapter will show how to know *for sure* if your baby is getting enough milk. If he isn't, the chapters that follow will guide you toward the steps to making more milk for your baby.

CHAPTER 3

How to Know If There Really Is a Problem

Before tackling the question of why your baby is not getting enough milk or deciding what to do about it, *you have to know for sure that there really is a problem.* This includes finding out approximately how much milk your baby is getting and whether it is enough for good growth, because the amount each baby needs to grow appropriately can vary. When you have the facts, you can build the best strategy for your specific situation.

Determining If Your Baby Is Getting Enough Milk

Because the breast does not have measurement marks like a bottle, you can't easily see how much milk baby is taking during feedings. Normally that's fine; when everything is going well, you don't need to know exactly how much he gets. But if you're worried, the best way to know is diaper output and weight gain.

Doctors look at many factors, but baby's weight gain usually is the bottom line. Between doctor visits, monitoring diaper output is normally sufficient because what is coming out is usually an indication of what is going in. If baby is gaining well, he should be having adequate diaper output; if he isn't, he won't. If his diaper output is high but his weight gain is low, then there is reason for

Adequate Milk Intake Criteria for Exclusively Breastfed Babies

Yes No

☐ ☐ Baby regains birth weight by two weeks of age.

☐ ☐ Between days two and three, baby's stools change from black to green and then turn to yellow, with "seeds" or "curds" by day five.

☐ ☐ After day four, baby has at least three stools per day that are bigger than a U.S. or Canadian quarter (2.5 cm) (*after the first four to six weeks, stools may be less frequent but are larger in size*).

☐ ☐ After day four or twenty-four hours after your milk comes in, baby has at least five very wet diapers that are odorless and colorless (*four wet diapers may be adequate if they are heavily soaked*).

☐ ☐ After day four or when milk is in, baby gains weight at the following *average* rate:

First three months: approximately 1 oz (30 g) per day or 6 oz (180 g) per week

Four to six months: at least 0.6 oz (18 g) per day

Seven to nine months: at least 0.4 oz (12 g) per day

Ten to twelve months: at least 0.3 oz (9 g) per day

☐ ☐ Optional: Feeding test weights indicate baby is getting enough milk (see "Feeding Test Weights," later in this chapter).

Sources: Nommsen-Rivers L, Heinig J, Cohen R, Dewey K. Newborn wet and soiled diaper counts and timing of onset of lactation as indicators of breast-feeding inadequacy. *J Hum Lact.* 2008;24(1):27–33. Dewey K, Nommsen-Rivers L, Heinig M, Cohen R. Risk factors for suboptimal infant breastfeeding behavior, delayed onset of lactation, and excess neonatal weight loss. *Pediatrics.* 2003;112(3 Pt 1):607–19.

further medical investigation. Beyond the first few days of birth, diaper output and weight gain or loss usually go hand in hand.

This chapter explains the fine points of measuring intake by weight gain and diaper output. The preceding checklist provides the minimum benchmarks of both weight gain and diaper output for an *exclusively* breastfed baby to grow adequately according to his age. Read through them and decide whether or not each statement is true for your baby.

Weight Gain to Gauge Milk Intake

When accurately measured, weight gain is the best indicator that your baby is getting enough milk. For this reason, obtaining an accurate weight each time is crucial when baby's intake is in question. Pay attention to these five factors:

1. **Accurate Readings.** Human error in taking weights is surprisingly common. The scale can be used incorrectly, the weight reading can be misread, the numbers can be transposed, the wrong weight can be recorded, or the percentile can be plotted incorrectly. To minimize errors, watch the reading being taken and double-check the figure yourself against what is written and plotted in your baby's chart.
2. **Scale Accuracy.** Weighings on different scales can yield different results because all scales are calibrated differently. Scale type also matters; electronic scales are more accurate than spring-loaded scales. Whichever is used, *comparing weights taken on the exact same scale gives the most accurate results.* If desired, you can rent a high-accuracy electronic scale from a pump rental station. The instant feedback of a home scale can be empowering because you'll know sooner if baby isn't gaining enough, avoiding the need for frequent doctor visits. Just remember that readings on your scale and your doctor's scale may not match.
3. **Clothing Removal.** Be sure to remove all clothing, including hat, socks, booties, and mittens. Don't forget to take off the diaper, too.
4. **Consistent Time Intervals.** The interval between readings should be as consistent as possible, even down to the time of day.

5. **Baby's Stomach and Colon Contents.** Accuracy can be further increased by timing the weights for after a bowel movement and before a feed.

Newborns may lose up to 7 percent of their birth weight in the first days after birth before they begin gaining. Occasionally, excessive weight loss (more than 10 percent) occurs rapidly even though baby appears to be nursing well. In some of these cases, it is believed that baby's birth weight may have been artificially inflated by extra water acquired during labor as the result of mother's IV fluids or medications. After birth, baby urinates the extra fluid. When excessive weight loss occurs together with multiple wet diapers in the first days after birth, this noncritical cause should be considered.

If your baby appears to be feeding well and is healthy, alert, and passing black, tarry meconium stools, chances are good that everything is fine and he will start gaining once milk production kicks into high gear. This means that if your milk "comes in" on the second day, he'll probably start gaining very early. But if it doesn't come in right away, he may lose a little more until milk production picks up. When milk is slow to come in and low intake becomes a problem, temporary supplementation may be needed.

Breastfed babies who are doing well often regain birth weight by the end of the first week. But because some mothers and babies may get a slower start, doctors usually are satisfied if baby regains his birth weight by the end of two weeks. Weighing him every few days or once a week is usually enough, but daily weighing may be necessary in critical cases.

But what if baby was gaining well in the early weeks or months and faltered only later on? It's OK for him to be on the lower end of the growth chart, but a significant *drop* in percentiles (such as having been in the seventieth percentile then dropping to the fiftieth) is cause for concern and further investigation.

Diaper Output to Gauge Milk Intake

In the first forty-eight hours (days one to two) after birth, an exclusively breastfed newborn will pass meconium stools and wet one or two diapers with pale yellow urine per day. Stools will lighten and turn greenish around day three. Reddish "brick dust" urine from uric acid crystals occasionally occurs before the milk comes in well but should be gone by the fourth to fifth day.

By day four (the fourth twenty-four-hour period), the milk is usually in, and meconium should transition to brownish-green and then yellow, while the urine should be nearly colorless and odorless. If your baby is still passing black or brown stools after the fourth day, this indicates low intake.

After the first six to eight weeks, the frequency of wet diapers may decrease, but they are heavier as baby's bladder grows. Bowel movements may continue to be frequent, or they may slow down to once a day or once every two or three days. A few babies may go once a week or even longer. You'll know if this is normal or not by the size and consistency of the stool. When a thriving baby's stooling pattern changes, the stools are still loose but proportionally larger. If you find yourself changing "blow-out" diapers every few days, chances are he's doing just fine.

In most cases, stool output is more important than urine output because babies who are not getting enough milk may be taking

How Wet Is "Very Wet"?

If you aren't sure what a "very wet" diaper feels like, take a fresh diaper and pour 2 tablespoons of water (1 ounce or 30 milliliters) on it; this is what a very wet diaper feels like. If baby weighs more than 8 pounds (3,636 grams), use 3 tablespoons of water (1.5 ounces or 45 milliliters). Save this sample in a sealed plastic bag to compare with baby's wet diapers.

in enough to urinate frequently but not enough to gain weight and produce enough stools. When in doubt, baby's weight can be checked to verify if there is any cause for concern.

A simple diaper chart can be a useful tool when you're not sure if your baby is getting enough. It helps you see at a glance if output is sufficient and sounds an early warning if things are not going well. A customizable chart is downloadable from www.lowmilksupply .org/chart, or you can make one yourself. You may find it convenient to put the chart on a clipboard above the baby's changing table.

Feeding Test Weights

It is possible to determine fairly closely how much milk your baby receives at a given breastfeeding by performing a test weight.[1] This technique is used by many lactation consultants and is especially useful in determining how much baby is getting at breast when he is also being supplemented, because diaper output and weight gain can't give you the full picture. It can also help determine how much to supplement (see Chapter 4).

To obtain a test weight, you'll need to rent a high-accuracy scale such as the Medela BabyWeigh or the Tanita BLB-12 or BD-815U. Weigh your baby before feeding him and record the weight, and then feed your baby as you normally would. *Don't change baby's diaper or clothing in any way.* When the feeding is complete, weigh your baby again. Subtract the first weight reading from the second; the difference is the amount of milk your baby took. Some scales have special functions that automatically calculate the weight difference.

Weight Conversions

Ounces can be measured in both weight and liquid volume. One ounce (weight) = 28.3495231 grams, and 1 ounce (liquid volume) = 29.5735297 milliliters. But for our purposes, it is easier and acceptable to use 1 ounce (weight) = 30 grams and 1 ounce (liquid volume) = 30 milliliters.

While test weights are an accurate way to measure how much milk is transferred during a feeding, the information must be interpreted cautiously. Babies vary the amounts taken at different feedings and times of the day, so a single test weight provides only a snapshot of one feeding. The best way to get a true and accurate picture, though not always practical, is to do test weights for twenty-four hours.

Measuring Production by Pumping

Although not often necessary, a pumping test can determine more precisely how much milk you are making. Until recently, the method most commonly recommended was to pump for twenty-four hours instead of breastfeeding and measure the amount. A better method that provides information in only four hours rather than twenty-four was recently developed by researchers Ching Tat Lai, Post Grad Dip, M.Sc.; Thomas Hale, Ph.D.; Peter Hartmann, Ph.D.; and colleagues. While some argue that a pump does not always remove milk as effectively as a baby does, this method was found to be a close approximation of a mother's milk production when a hospital-grade pump is used. Because it interrupts breastfeeding, use this method only after exploring baby's milk intake and when the information gained outweighs the risks and expense.

> **Four-Hour Test:** Empty both breasts thoroughly once an hour for four hours with a high-grade pump (preferably hospital grade). Record the amounts of milk removed at hours three and four, then add them together and divide by two. The result is your average rate of milk production per hour. Multiply by twenty-four for your current daily milk production rate.[2]

The Final Results

You now have all the important facts to begin the process of understanding what is happening and what can be done about it. If your baby has numerous diapers and adequate weight gain, he's getting enough milk and all is well. Take a deep breath and *go enjoy your baby*. But if he still seems miserable or hungry, your doctor may need to rule out a physical problem. *Don't hesitate to seek a second opinion if you aren't satisfied with the answer and your gut feeling is that something is wrong*, even if that means asking the same doctor to reconsider. Once you both feel confident that there are no physical problems, there is the possibility that oversupply may be causing gassiness and pain (see Chapter 2). When no other reasons for your baby's fussiness can be found, the books *The Fussy Baby* by Dr. William Sears and *The No-Cry Sleep Solution* by Elizabeth Pantley can help you soothe your baby in ways that are supportive of breastfeeding.

If output and weight gain indicate that baby isn't getting enough milk yet you seem to have plenty, he may be unable to remove milk effectively, he may be self-limiting his feedings, or you may be having difficulties with milk ejection. Your milk production might be at risk, so while you figure out the problem, it's a good idea to pump, use breast compressions, or both. Chapter 7 discusses the types of difficulties that can prevent babies from feeding well despite an adequate milk supply. Chapter 8 addresses anatomical issues that can disrupt breastfeeding, and Chapter 10 describes ways milk ejection can be affected.

If your baby isn't getting enough milk, don't be discouraged. In many cases, milk production can be increased, depending on the reason that it's low. If the problem is the result of how breastfeed-

Find an IBCLC in Your Area

We maintain an international list of IBCLCs specializing in low milk supply on our website at www.lowmilksupply.org/lc.shtml, and there is a general list on the International Lactation Consultant Association (ILCA) website, www.ilca.org. Also, many U.S. Women, Infants, and Children (WIC) offices employ IBCLCs. Often, though, the best way to find an expert IBCLC is word of mouth. Ask your family, friends, obstetrician, and pediatrician.

ing has been managed, you may be able to solve it yourself with the information provided in this book. If the problem stems from an issue with your breasts or hormones or is baby related, you will probably benefit from discussing what you learn with a lactation consultant, preferably one qualified to help mothers in challenging situations as an International Board Certified Lactation Consultant (IBCLC).

Developing a Milk Management Strategy

If you know for sure that your baby isn't getting enough of your milk, you'll need to develop a strategy for improving the situation. A good starting place are the three rules for solving breastfeeding problems taught by Kay Hoover, M.Ed., IBCLC, an author and lactation consultant in Pennsylvania:

> **Rule #1—Feed the Baby (Chapter 4):** A baby who is well fed will feed better at breast.
>
> **Rule #2—Protect the Milk Supply (Chapter 5):** Milk must be removed regularly and thoroughly to keep production as high as possible.
>
> **Rule #3—Find and Fix the Problem (Chapters 6 through 14):** When both baby and the milk supply are safe, you can then investigate the problem and develop a strategy to solve it.

Even though you may feel anxious to begin figuring out what the problem is and increasing your milk supply, your first priority is to make sure your baby is well fed. Supplementary feedings may be necessary, at least for a short time. The next chapter will help you determine the best way to give them in a way that supports breastfeeding.

Making the Most of What You Have

Emily's Story

Breastfeeding my baby Joshua was challenging. I had sore nipples and engorgement. He became jaundiced, and it was a constant battle to keep him awake. By three weeks of age, Joshua weighed nearly a pound (454 grams) less than when he was born. Not good.

The pediatricians wanted to see him every three days to monitor his weight, but their constantly changing advice was frustrating. Finally, when Joshua was five weeks old and still under birth weight, I was referred to a lactation consultant, who explained that I had less lactation tissue than normal. She gave me hope that I *could* continue to breastfeed. I started using a Lact-Aid® at-breast supplementer. It felt awkward and silly at first, but Joshua got all the food he needed. I usually nursed on both sides without the supplementer and then nursed with it to "top him off." Once he began eating solids, I nursed him without it. These were my happiest months as a nursing mother. Joshua breastfed until he was eleven months old.

My second son, Nathan, was born two years after Joshua. I felt much more confident with breastfeeding, but after ten days of exclusive nursing, Nathan hadn't gained any weight, so I started using the supplementer again. I was frustrated that I couldn't breastfeed exclusively but knew it would be OK. Like his brother, he breastfed for close to a year. My sons and I developed our own version of breastfeeding, and I am so grateful that we were persistent. There is something special in putting your child to your breast, even if you need a little bit of help.

CHAPTER 4

Supplementing Without Decreasing Your Milk Supply

Rule number one, while you're figuring out why your milk production is low and what you can do to improve it, is to make sure that your baby has enough to eat. Supplementation can seem like a step away from breastfeeding, but it really is a step forward, because it will ultimately help your baby be strong and able to breastfeed better. The next two chapters focus on ways to optimize your production. If baby needs more than he's been getting, this chapter will help you learn how to supplement without reducing supply or interfering with your developing breastfeeding relationship.

When to Begin Supplementation

The urgency to supplement depends on how much milk your baby is currently getting. The lower your baby's diaper output, weight gain, or feeding test weights, the more critical it is to begin supplementation immediately. On the other hand, if your baby's diaper output is borderline or just below minimum, weight gain is just below normal, or test weights are only slightly low, you may have more leeway in determining if, when, and how to give supplements. An otherwise healthy baby who is not getting quite enough because of something simple like infrequent nursing may be able to bring up your supply in a short amount of time without compromising his health.

How Much to Supplement: A Starting Point

Figuring out how much to supplement means finding the right balance between enough and not too much. Your baby needs sufficient food, but not so much that he feeds less often and understimulates your production. The following information is a *starting point* in determining how much to give. From there, you can customize it to your baby's needs.

Step One: Determine the Total Amount Needed

The first month is a time of rapid growth and building up of your milk production. By the end of that first month through at least the next five months, most babies are taking an average of about 25 ounces (750 milliliters) of milk per twenty-four hours. Babies under a month or who weigh less than 10 pounds (4,540 grams) often need less. An old rule of thumb is about 2.5 ounces (75 milliliters) of milk for every pound (454 grams) of body weight per twenty-four hours. Divide the total amount needed each day by the average number of feedings per day to determine the average amount baby needs at each feeding. If your starting point is 25 ounces, the milk calculator at www.kellymom.com/bf/pumping/milkcalc.html illustrates high and low ranges.

Step Two: Determine the Amount of Supplement Needed

If you've taken test weights and have an idea of the average amount baby is getting from you each feeding (Chapter 3), subtract it from the total amount you determined baby requires each feeding. The result is the average amount of supplement needed per feeding. For example, if you know that your six-week-old baby feeds about eight times a day and needs about 3 ounces per feeding but has been getting only 2 ounces at the breast, you can probably expect him to want an additional ounce per feeding.

If you don't have a good idea of what baby has been getting, take baby's weight gain deficit for the previous week and then multiply it by 2 for the ounces of total extra milk he may need per twenty-four hours. So if baby should be gaining 7 ounces a week but gained only 2 the previous week, then he may need 10 ounces of supplement (5 ounces × 2) per day to start.

Once you've found your starting point, offer this amount and watch carefully to see if baby wants less or more. Give him whatever he will take, but don't ask him to take more than he really wants. Keep in mind that babies, like adults, vary in how much food they want from one feeding to the next. Estimating the amount of extra milk needed is as much an art as it is a science, and baby himself needs to play a role in this process. If he seems ravenous and he wasn't feeding too quickly, don't hesitate to give him a little more than you planned. The key to making adjustments lies in balancing three factors: (1) good diaper output, (2) appropriate weight gain, and (3) baby's satisfaction. Adjust the amount you offer up or down a half ounce at a time unless it's obvious that your estimate was really far off. If the change works, stay with it until it isn't working, and then adjust again.

The Significantly Underfed Baby

While we usually trust babies to tell us how much food they need, some circumstances do require parents to take over for a while. A seriously underfed baby (who may have misled you with his passive behavior) may not show strong hunger cues or may quit nursing before he has had enough. His diaper output and weight gain are poor, and his feeding behavior may be lethargic. Giving him at least a half ounce by bottle or another method prior to breastfeeding can energize him to feed better. Or he may simply need to be fed in whatever way it takes to get enough milk into him until he is stronger.

Once they start really eating, underweight babies frequently want more than the usual amount while they catch up on their

Supplementation at Night

At first, you may need to offer supplements at every feeding, including nighttime. Later, when your baby has begun gaining well or he is older and able to go longer between feedings, it may be possible to forgo supplementing at night.

weight. This usually slows down once baby reaches the weight he should be based on his birth weight and current age. At-breast supplementation, as described later in this chapter, is not a good choice until baby grows stronger. Be sure to pump after breastfeeding to ensure thorough drainage.

Choosing a Supplement

According to the World Health Organization, the best supplement is expressed milk from baby's own mother, followed by pasteurized human donor milk, and then commercially synthesized infant milk (formula). Consult with your baby's pediatrician to determine which is most appropriate for your situation. More information about supplementation options is available on our website.

If you're making plenty of milk but baby is having difficulty getting it out, you should be able to provide everything he needs by pumping. But if baby needs formula, first offer whatever you can express—no amount is too small. It's preferable to give your milk separately to ensure that baby gets every precious drop and none is thrown out because he didn't finish a supplement combined with your milk.

Supplementation Devices

There are many devices that can be used to feed supplementary milk to your baby, including at-breast supplementers, bottles, finger-feeders, cups, eyedroppers, medicine droppers, and syringes. Each has advantages and disadvantages, and you may decide to use

Pasteurizing Human Milk

The U.S. Centers for Disease Control and Prevention recommend against informally donated human milk because of the risk of transmitting harmful bacteria or viruses, but some mothers prefer to use milk from a trusted friend or relative when banked milk is not an option. Heat-treating the milk first can minimize any risks.[1]

Containers for storing your milk should be washed and clean, but they don't need to be sterilized. First, place about 2 to 5 ounces (60 to 150 milliliters) of milk in a pint-sized (450 milliliter) covered glass jar and set aside. Then bring about 2 cups (450 milliliters) of water to a boil in a small pot. Turn off the heat and place the jar in the water for twenty minutes. When the milk is cool, it can be fed to baby. Treated milk should be stored in the same sealed container that it was pasteurized in to avoid bacterial contamination. It can be kept safely at room temperature for up to eight hours and refrigerated for up to twelve.

different devices at different stages as circumstances change. Some work best when you have a skilled consultant to teach you the little tricks of the trade that you may need and how to avoid the pitfalls that could sabotage your success. No matter which supplementation device you choose, incorporate as much feeding at the breast as possible to maximize milk removal, minimize flow preference, and maintain baby's familiarity with the breast.

At-Breast Supplementers

At-breast supplementers use a receptacle to contain milk and a plastic tube to carry milk to the mother's nipple, where baby can draw from it as he nurses. They are especially appropriate when low milk production is due to maternal causes. At-breast supplementers also can be used for some infant-related situations as long as the baby is able to draw enough milk out in a reasonable amount of time. There are commercial products such as the Medela SNS™ (Supplemental Nursing System), Ameda Breastfeeding Aid™, and

Lact-Aid. Or, a 3.5 or 5 French gavage tube can also be used by attaching it to a syringe or threading it into a regular baby bottle with a slightly enlarged nipple hole and submerging the end of the tubing in the milk. Detailed information about the different at-breast supplementers and tips for using them can be found at www .lowmilksupply.org/abs.shtml.

At-breast supplementers can be awkward to manage with newborns who have difficulty latching. An alternative is to use a Monoject 412 periodontal syringe commonly used by dentists, which has a nicely curved hard tip instead of a needle. Baby first latches to the breast, and then the plastic tip of the syringe is gently sneaked into the corner of his mouth no more than an eighth to a quarter of an inch (two and a half to five millimeters). As he sucks, the plunger is depressed with short taps to deliver small amounts of milk whenever baby's jaw drops. Several syringes can be prepared for a feeding so that they can easily be switched out to maintain a constant flow. Since they hold a small amount and last only about a week, syringes may not be practical for long-term use.

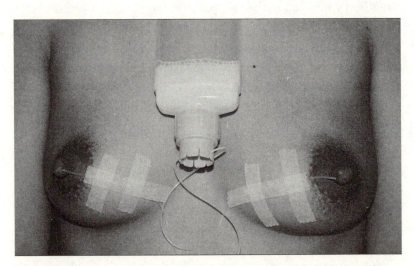

This at-breast supplementer tubing has been placed to enter the lower part of baby's mouth when he is held across the lap and to stop short of the nipple so baby doesn't use it like a straw.

Not all mothers feel entirely comfortable with these devices. For some, it is a blatant reminder that they don't have enough milk and need a "prosthesis" in order to breastfeed. More effort is required to prepare, set up, and clean them than regular bottles, and it can take a few days or even weeks to become proficient and feel comfortable using them. At-breast supplementers can leak if not properly assembled and aren't as discreet for public nursing. However, many mothers overcome these challenges and say they feel more like a regular breastfeeding mother because the entire feeding is at breast and they prefer the intimacy it allows to other methods.

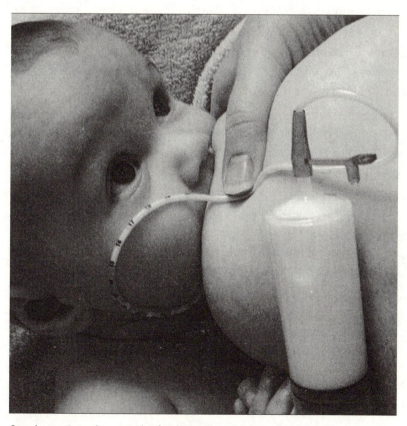

Supplementing at breast with a feeding tube and syringe combination

Bottles

The upside of bottles is that they are easy, convenient, and socially acceptable. The downside is that there is a risk of nipple confusion and flow preference that could jeopardize your breastfeeding relationship. However, there are ways that bottles can be used to support breastfeeding and reduce these risks.

Nipple confusion and flow preference are two very different problems. Debra Swank, IBCLC, explains that *nipple confusion* happens when a baby given an artificial nipple or pacifier forgets how to breastfeed. He starts to root for the breast but either can't latch or doesn't move his tongue correctly when he does latch. This occurs more commonly in newborns who have had only limited opportunities to nurse and received a bottle before imprinting upon the breast. When babies arch, cry, scream, or otherwise actively push away the breast, or simply turn away in quiet disinterest after exposure to bottles, it may be due to *flow preference*. Once a baby has become accustomed to the instant gratification of a bottle that flows immediately and never stops until it's empty, it can be harder for the breast to compete when it doesn't flow until mother has a milk ejection and then does so in spurts according to baby's demand. This can be worsened when milk production is decreased.

Nipple preference can happen when there is a significant mismatch between the mother's nipple shape and the shape of the artificial nipple. For instance, when a mother has very small nipples that protrude only slightly and the artificial nipple is large and long and easier to grasp, baby may prefer the more prominent artificial nipple.

When choosing an artificial nipple for bottle supplementation, look for one that approximates breastfeeding by encouraging baby to latch deeply, extend his tongue, and cup it around the nipple with relaxed lips. Ultrasound studies show that round nipples with a broad base encourage these motions.[2] Although flattened-tip orthodontic nipples are often recommended, babies tend to retract their tongues while sucking on them, the opposite of what should happen on the breast. In addition to reducing milk transfer, this type of tongue movement can cause abraded, sore nipples when baby breastfeeds.

The most important factor in minimizing flow preference is slowing the flow rate of the bottle. Look for slow-flowing nipples; they are usually labeled "slow-flow" or "newborn." Not all nipples are created equal. You can test and compare them by turning them upside down and seeing how fast milk drips out. Check those you select periodically as well, since they can wear out and flow more rapidly over time. Products that use an inner chamber to regulate flow seem to help ease the transition to the breast. Babies respond differently to various nipples, so it may take some trial and error to find the best one for your baby. Since the flow from your breast doesn't tend to increase over time, slow-flow nipples will continue to be best even when baby gets older.

Bottle-Feeding Methods That Minimize Flow Preference. You can help baby maintain or learn breastfeeding behaviors while he feeds from the bottle by teaching him to take it in a way that is similar to how he latches to the breast. Instead of "poking" the nipple in his half-opened mouth, offer it pointed up toward the ceiling and touch or stroke the side downward across his lips. This eventually triggers a wide gape, like a yawn. Then move the *base* of the nipple to his lower lip and roll it downward into his mouth so that he takes it in deeply. Holding baby upright with the bottle parallel with the floor can further reduce the flow. Despite marketing efforts to convince you otherwise, there is no need to keep the nipple full of milk, nor is swallowing air an issue because air tends to come right back up naturally as baby burps.

Babies feed better when bottle feedings are periodically paused, or *paced*, simulating the way that breastfeeding babies slow down in between milk ejections. After a few minutes of sucking, or if you see baby's forehead and eyes show signs of stress, tip him forward gently until the milk runs out of the nipple, without removing the nipple from his mouth. This helps baby retain control of the feeding, reminds him to stop when he is full, and helps him to better coordinate sucking, swallowing, and breathing.

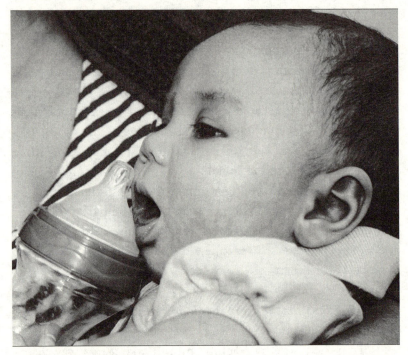

Latching a bottle deeply

When to Offer the Bottle. Traditional wisdom says that bottles should be given only after offering the breast so that baby sucks actively to remove the most milk. However, a hungry baby may have less patience for a breast with low supply and may stop trying without taking all the milk that's there. It's as if they know the bottle is coming and are just "paying their dues" at breast. As a result, they take increasing amounts by bottle, and milk production slows down, requiring even more supplements. This downward spiral effect is the reason that supplementing by bottle has such a poor reputation.

Christina Smillie, M.D., IBCLC, suggests an alternative way that she calls the "Finish at the Breast" method of bottle supplementation. In her practice, she observed that babies who quenched their initial hunger and thirst with a bottle first tended to have more patience feeding at the breast. She began suggesting that mothers give a *limited* amount of supplement *before* breastfeeding and discovered that babies would breastfeed longer even if the flow was slow, removing more milk and increasing milk production.

Another great aspect of the "Finish at the Breast" method is that baby learns to associate the euphoria of fullness with the breast rather than the bottle, while you get the satisfaction of a contented, "milk drunk" baby falling asleep at your breast. When it happens the other way around, it can be disheartening and undermine your confidence to the point that you end up breastfeeding less and less.

The key to this technique is giving about one-fourth to one-half ounce (7 to 15 milliliters) *less* by bottle than the amount your baby usually needs or takes. If too much is given, baby will not be hungry enough to feed well or long enough at breast. If too little is given, he may not have the patience to nurse. When he looks relaxed or finishes the bottle, whichever comes first, switch to the breast. If he fusses and seems to want more supplement after breastfeeding, give it to him, but be sure to finish at the breast, even if for just a minute or two. It may take a few days of trial and error to determine the best amount.

Be flexible and watch baby's body language so you can respond to the normal fluctuations in your production. You may find, for example, that you can give fewer supplements (or none!) during the night and before the morning feedings, but in the late afternoon or early evening, you need to give more. This is fine when it follows the normal fluctuations in your milk supply. As your supply increases, you'll be able to decrease the amount offered up front, little by little. The degree to which this method can increase milk production depends on the reason it is low. If the cause is secondary, it is likely to respond better to this technique than if the cause is primary. But either way, this method can work well to encourage baby to breastfeed as much and as effectively as possible.

Breast Refusal. If baby begins to show signs of breast refusal, *don't* think he is rejecting you as his mother or that it's permanent. It just means that conditions need to change to make feeding at the breast more desirable. A baby who has experienced milk flowing more easily from the bottle may not trust the breast, even when milk production is improved. He has found something that works for him, so why change? Increasing milk production and flow is helpful, but regaining baby's trust takes time and a gentle approach. Efforts to woo him back to the breast can be draining, and you may question whether it is right to "force the issue." But in this case, your baby doesn't know what is best for him—you do. A gentle approach will work better than trying to impose your will on your baby. You may have to work slowly and help him make the transition in stages. Giving the bottle with baby turned toward the breast or with a cheek on your bare breast can help build more positive associations. You can also try placing the bottle under your armpit, preferably by a bare breast, so that baby must face you more fully when he feeds from the bottle as he would at the breast. Offering the breast when he is sleepy and placing him upright skin to skin to take advantage of his nursing instincts can also help baby overcome his resistance. Once he begins latching, he'll gradually learn to trust the breast again over several feedings or days, and then feedings will become the enjoyable experience that they were meant to be. If nothing seems to work, a lactation consultant may have more ideas using methods that tap into his natural reflexes.

Finger-Feeding

If baby must be fed away from the breast and you don't want to use a bottle, finger-feeding is another option. This avoids the use of an artificial nipple and may be especially useful for babies who have certain types of suck problems. A finger-feeder can be made at home using the same gavage tube system described previously. The Hazelbaker FingerFeeder™ is a commercial finger-feeding device. You can also use an at-breast supplementer clipped to clothing or hung around the neck as usual, with the tubing attached to a finger.

As with using a bottle, it is important to encourage your baby to open his mouth widely before the finger is offered so that he learns the same skills he needs for breastfeeding. Some lactation consultants also recommend using the finger or thumb that is closest to the approximate diameter of your nipple.

Monoject 412 periodontal syringes with a curved hard tip instead of a needle are another option for finger-feeding. They hold from one-third to one-half ounce of liquid and are inexpensive (about US$1.00). Those with larger barrels usually give too much milk with even a small push, while smaller ones simply may not hold enough milk. Finger-feeding with a syringe is "parent led" rather than "baby led," allowing more parental control over milk flow. This can be an advantage for babies who have trouble drawing the milk out of feeding tubes. Eye and medicine droppers have also been used to finger-feed but do not offer as much control over how much milk is coming out.

Important Note: Finger-feeding is great in the right circumstances, but if done incorrectly or at the wrong time, it can cause problems as well. For best results, have a skilled lactation consultant teach and observe you; their input is a worthwhile investment. More information on finger-feeding can be found at www .lowmilksupply.org.

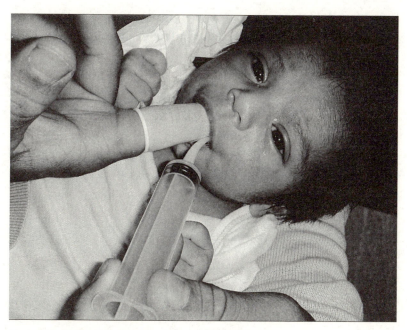

Finger-feeding with a periodontal syringe (glove optional)

Cups

Although you might think that drinking from a cup is an advanced skill beyond the capability of infants, babies as young as thirty weeks gestation have been successfully cup-fed, sometimes before they can effectively breastfeed or bottle-feed. Cup-feeding supports breast-feeding by avoiding nipple or flow preference. However, there can be significant spillage, which can be frustrating and expensive.

Almost any clean, small plastic or glass cup or bowl can be used to cup-feed, with the exception of disposal paper cups that may contain a plastic coating toxic to infants. There are also cups specially designed for feeding small babies, such as the Medela Soft-Feeder™ and Baby Cup Feeder™, the Ameda Baby Cup™, and the Foley Cup Feeder. The Medela SoftFeeder and the Foley Cup Feeder work especially well because they feature a small self-filling reservoir that allows control over the flow of supplement. For more information on how to cup-feed, visit www.lowmilksupply.org.

Weaning from Supplements

If your milk production increases significantly and baby begins consistently refusing supplement while continuing to gain well, then it is time to stop supplementing. Test weights can confirm that he is getting the amount he needs, or you can just monitor his diaper output and weight gain.

If baby is not yet refusing supplements but your milk supply seems to be increasing or he begins to gain more quickly than necessary, try decreasing the supplement by one-fourth to one-half ounce (7 to 15 milliliters) per feed every few days. You may need to go more slowly, or you may not be able to go lower. Never stop supplementing abruptly if your milk production is not adequate to replace the supplementary feedings.

Solids as Supplements

The introduction of solids around the middle of baby's first year is an important milestone. While the first amounts of solid foods babies eat are usually small, about a teaspoon (5 milliliters or 4.7 grams) per meal, starting solids marks the end of baby's complete nutritional dependence on your milk or formula. It is often at this point that mothers are able to gradually replace supplemental feedings with solid foods. However, be sure that solid foods replace supplements, not your milk.

CHAPTER 5

Getting Your Milk Supply Off to a Good Start

As a pregnant or new mother, you may be concerned about making enough milk because of previous supply problems, breast surgery, hormonal problems, or a family history of problems. But before diving into how to increase your milk, let's talk about some of the things you can do to lay a foundation for the best possible start from pregnancy onward.

Get a Head Start: Expressing Milk Before Baby Is Born

Sue Cox, AM, RM, IBCLC, a midwife and lactation consultant in Australia, recommends an old method that seems to help get things going: removing colostrum during late pregnancy.[1] This method has not been validated scientifically, but at least it can provide colostrum for any supplementation that's needed. Concern is occasionally voiced that prenatal milk expression could stimulate labor prematurely, but there is no research supporting this, and in fact, women have safely nursed during pregnancy throughout time.[2] Unless you are at high risk, this practice seems to be safe for most mothers.

Begin hand expressing daily starting at the thirty-fourth week of pregnancy when you're relaxed and warm, such as after taking a hot shower. (Stop if you have any unusually strong contractions.) Express any colostrum drops into a spoon, then use a small periodontal or similar blunt-end syringe to draw it up. You can refrigerate and reuse the same syringe for forty-eight hours, adding more colostrum as it is expressed, then freeze it in an airtight zip-close bag for the hospital.

A variation on this idea is practiced in some cultures. Young husbands are taught that it is their duty to suckle their wives' breasts during lovemaking in preparation for future babies. Some lactation consultants report that these first-time mothers seem to experience early and abundant milk production. If your partner is so inclined, it may be worth trying.

Nurse in the First Hour

Ideally, breastfeeding should begin as soon after birth as possible, when the baby is ready to nurse. When placed on their mothers' bare abdomen immediately after birth, most newborns will find the breast and initiate suckling in fewer than fifty minutes.[3] They seem to be able to get more colostrum during this golden time, possibly due to oxytocin from labor also affecting the breast. Separating an infant from his mother during this crucial alert period misses his first opportunity to begin breastfeeding using his instinctual abilities. Instead, he may pass to the resting phase, becoming too drowsy to try much during the next several hours. Ensuring that your baby has every opportunity to suckle right after birth will help you get a great start on your milk production. So long as baby is healthy and there are no pressing medical concerns, don't be afraid to tell anyone who might suggest he needs to be bathed or measured or anything else that you are keeping him with you for the time being. Those things can be done later. Smile, be polite, and be firm. It's *your* baby, not the hospital's!

But what if you don't have that ideal birth? If baby has any health concerns, you may not be able to spend that first hour cuddling. Even when given the opportunity, some babies don't seem able to latch well immediately after delivery. This is often the result of mother's labor drugs, including epidurals, that cross the placenta and affect the baby in varying degrees. Most types can temporarily diminish an infant's spontaneous breast-seeking and nursing behaviors, and some also increase body temperature and crying.[4] However, not being able to nurse the baby right after birth does not doom you to trouble; it just means that it may take a little more work to get breastfeeding started.

Mothers who have cesarean births (C-sections) should be able to nurse a healthy infant with no complications while in the recovery room after surgery. Most of these babies do well, though some may be sleepier and less interested in nursing if you labored for some time with medications or received general anesthesia. Urgent cesarean births have been associated with delayed milk production, possibly related to the stress involved.[5] However, lots of skin-to-skin contact and frequent nursing as soon as is practical will go a long way toward minimizing potential problems. It may be reassuring to know that most mothers who have had cesarean births have good milk supplies.

If you and baby are separated after birth or baby is unable to breastfeed, try to hand express or pump within the first hour after birth and at least every three hours thereafter until baby is able to begin nursing. Not only will you get more colostrum for any supplement baby needs, but expressing when your body expects it to be removed yields more and also helps to jump-start the milk production process.

Keep Baby Skin to Skin as Much as Possible

One of the most enjoyable and beneficial things you can do as a mother is simply holding your baby "skin to skin." With baby wearing only a diaper and your bra removed, snuggle him upright, nestled between your breasts. Your breasts will actually heat up or cool down in response to your baby's body temperature, but if needed, a blanket can be placed around the two of you. This kind of skin-to-skin contact has been shown to help increase milk volume.[6] An additional benefit is that baby is also more likely to nurse when he is "in the restaurant" and smelling your milk.

Delay Bathing

Baby may show more interest in breastfeeding if you delay bathing him until he has had some skin-to-skin time with you. If there are any problems, consider postponing a shower yourself for a day or two. Babies who are placed on their mothers' chests with their hands free after birth smear amniotic fluid onto the breasts as they use their hands and face to find them. Later, the smell of the fluid seems to draw them to the breast like a tracking beacon.[7] This biological sequence helps babies cue into their natural latching instincts.

Optimal Milk Production Depends on an Optimal Latch

Your baby's ability to get all the milk available is strongly dependent on how well he is attached to the breast. If he doesn't latch effectively, he cannot remove milk well from the breast. Ideas about *how* to get baby to attach well to the breast have been evolving in recent years. The basic objective is to get the mother's breast and nipple positioned deeply in the baby's mouth. At one time, it seemed that lactation counselors believed that there was only one right way to do this and that a mother must follow the "correct" procedure, like a recipe. Today, skilled counselors understand that there is no single correct way for a baby to latch to the breast. The only essential measures of a good latch are that mother and baby are comfortable and that milk transfers efficiently. Great books for understanding how baby can latch more effectively include *Breast-*

feeding Made Simple by Nancy Mohrbacher, IBCLC, and Kathleen Kendall-Tackett, Ph.D., IBCLC, and *The Latch* by Jack Newman, M.D., IBCLC, and Teresa Pitman. We also provide a detailed explanation on our website at www.lowmilksupply.org/latch.

Once baby latches, pay close attention to how it feels. It's normal to feel some tenderness in the early days, but if it actually hurts, he is probably latched too shallowly. Encourage a deeper latch by changing your position or the way he comes to the breast. If the pain continues, something is wrong no matter how good the latch may look on the outside; seek help from a lactation consultant sooner rather than later.

If baby isn't latching successfully by the end of the first six hours, keep him skin to skin to stimulate his feeding reflexes and begin expressing colostrum. Don't use your pump quite yet, though; hand expression usually gets more out than a pump in the beginning (see the video: newborns.stanford.edu/Breastfeeding/HandExpression.html). It also works well if your breasts become uncomfortably full as the milk comes in because pumping can draw more fluid into your areolas, which causes swelling and makes

Is Frequent Nursing the First Three Days a Bad Sign?

During the first three days after birth, many babies will nurse quite voraciously until full milk production starts. Nursing sessions can feel like marathons and last up to several hours off and on, without any clear beginning or end. You may wonder if baby will ever come up for air! Rest assured that this doesn't mean baby needs more than you are making right now. A newborn's stomach is very small at birth and stretches out gradually over the first week as your milk comes in. An extra hungry baby simply helps to hasten the increase in milk volume, but at a pace that is healthy for him.

latching difficult for your baby. Before pumps were invented, women throughout time have hand expressed very effectively. Try expressing a few drops of colostrum onto a plastic spoon for someone else to offer the baby while you express into a second spoon.

If you can't express much colostrum in the first few days, it doesn't mean that it isn't there. Swollen breast tissue caused by water retention after birth can make expressing colostrum or milk difficult the first few days, and hand expression is a skill that takes some practice. Colostrum, which can be golden or clear like saliva, is produced in very small quantities. Babies take on average about 1 to 3 teaspoons (5 to 15 milliliters) per feeding, but every drop is valuable.

Optimizing Milk Removal: Breast Massage and Compression

Once baby is latching well, maximizing drainage helps strengthen the signal to make more milk. One of the difficulties of low milk production is that milk ejection is often less effective when it has less volume to work with, so milk may not be completely drained by the baby or a pump. To get the most milk out, massage your breasts both before and during feeding (or pumping). One study looked at the effect of simultaneous massage with pumping and found 40 to 50 percent more milk was removed when pumping with massage than without it.[8]

One popular variation of breast massage is called *breast compression* and uses external hand pressure to push out any residual milk. Hold your breast with your thumb on top and your fingers underneath (or vice versa), far back on the breast away from the areola. Compress the tissue between your fingers and thumb gently but firmly—it shouldn't hurt or pinch ducts—and hold the compression. If you feel any firm or lumpy areas, focus your efforts there as they may contain pockets of milk. Baby usually will begin swallowing more rapidly, or you will see milk spraying into the pump flange. When baby's swallows or the milk spray slows, release

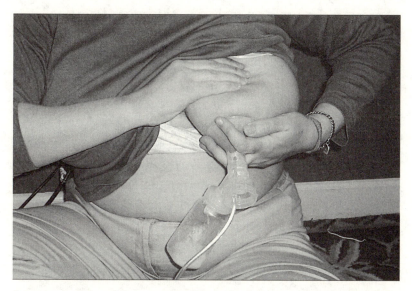

Breast compression while pumping and breastfeeding can increase the amount of milk removed.

the pressure and rotate a little to another firm area, repeating the process.

Proximity and Frequency

Research shows that there is no medical reason for healthy mothers and babies to be separated, which is why those central nurseries from our mothers' days are slowly being phased out. Staying in close proximity to your baby after birth stimulates him to feed more often and helps you to respond to his earliest hunger cues. So nurse, nurse, and nurse some more, *at least* eight times each twenty-four hours for as long as baby desires. Remember that frequent feedings in the early days are normal, and for mothers at risk of low milk production, they may be essential to calibrate the highest milk supply possible. They also help create greater storage capacity, which allows you to store more milk at one time for baby. In general, the best way to make *more* milk is to *take* more milk.

Worried About Becoming a "Human Pacifier"?

Letting baby nurse when he isn't actively feeding or for comfort between feedings isn't wrong. It won't cause bad habits or an unhealthy dependence on the breast. *Pacifiers are artificial replacements for your breasts, the original place of comfort.* Babies nurse for many reasons besides hunger. There is great comfort when nursing at your breast, nuzzling close to your body, smelling your familiar smells, and being held in your loving arms. Decades of child development research have shown that a baby whose needs are met learns trust and security. Listen to your maternal instinct; nature gave it to you for a reason because it prompts you to give your baby what he needs to survive and thrive.

Avoid the Visitor Syndrome

Those well-meaning relatives and friends arrive at your hospital room with great excitement, forgetting that you are just learning how to breastfeed. Some mothers then give bottles of formula because they're uncomfortable nursing or pumping in front of others or asking them to leave. The *visitor syndrome* can continue at home as friends and family show up to see the new little one. Some mothers feel obligated to stay with their visitors, especially those from out of town. Well-meaning friends and relatives may ask to feed baby a bottle or suggest that the baby isn't hungry yet, he just needs to be held . . . or given a pacifier . . . or walked . . . or burped . . . anything but put back to the breast, because it is surely too soon. By the time everyone leaves, you're exhausted, baby's frazzled, and breastfeeding is off to a slow start. Remember that nursing your baby is ultimately more important than your visitors' feelings. Feel free to reclaim your motherhood by assertively asking for the time and space you need to concentrate on caring for your baby.

Express Milk After Breastfeeding

The first few weeks are an opportunity to maximize your milk-making potential by removing additional milk after or between as many feedings as you can. This will calibrate your production as high as possible. Once your milk comes in, a pump can assist you in this job. Although you may have purchased or received a consumer-grade pump before baby was born, they are designed for moms who have established milk supplies and are using them two to four times a day while at work or school. Hospital-grade pumps are heavier duty and best for maximizing milk removal at this critical time in building your milk production.

Pumping for a few minutes after as many feedings as possible (unless baby is nursing *really* often and effectively) should continue for at least the first three weeks and then until you are sure your baby is getting enough milk. If the diaper count is low and baby needs supplementation, be sure to feed him any milk you express. Chapter 11 discusses pumping in more detail.

Don't Skip Nighttime Feedings

Most mothers willingly feed their babies whenever necessary during the daytime but find themselves longing for an uninterrupted night's sleep. At the same time, newborns often sleep longer during the daytime and eat more at night. Temptation may loom large to avoid night feedings or to have someone else feed the baby while you sleep. But here's what you need to know: prolactin levels are higher at night when you sleep, and the prolactin surge in response to baby's suckling is also greater than in the daytime.[9] Milk flows more easily then because mother is sleepy and relaxed. This winning combination will go far in maximizing your milk production.

While it may seem that pumping during the daytime so someone else can give a bottle of pumped milk while you sleep is one way to have the best of both worlds, it can still cause your milk production to decrease because FIL builds up in the accumulating milk.

The first key to successful night nursing is to find a lying-down position (in a bed, not a reclining chair) that works for you and baby. While this comes easily for some mothers, it may take time and experimentation for others. Once this is accomplished, you may find yourself among the fortunate mothers who are able to doze right through feedings, especially when baby is a little older and can easily self-latch.

Second, take at least one or two naps during the daytime. They don't have to be long, but close your eyes and let yourself drift off once baby is asleep. Flow with baby's sleep pattern instead of resisting it; you will be surprised at how much this extra sleep can help. Even short naps cause prolactin to rise, once again giving you another hormonal boost. If you find it hard to nap because you have other young children or children who need care, this is the time to ask family and friends for help so you can get some rest.

Attitude is the final ingredient and plays the biggest role in how well rested mothers feel. Those who stress and resent nighttime feedings often wake up tired, grumpy, and irritable. Those who give themselves over to baby's temporary night needs, however, and who see this as a passing stage or a gift to their baby often find that they feel rested and able to function. In fact, they may not even remember how many times baby actually fed the night before. Your attitude, naps, and an early bedtime really can make a world of difference in how rested you feel.

Putting It All Together: The Essential Elements

Getting your milk production off to the very best start hinges on frequent and thorough drainage of the breasts from birth onward. With an optimal latch, baby will do his part to the best of his ability. All you need do is follow his lead and allow him to breastfeed whenever he asks. Having realistic expectations of new mother-hood and a plan to nurture yourself will also help you to cope and even flourish during this time. Preparation and making baby your first priority will help you to maximize your milk-making potential now and eliminate the most common causes of low milk production.

Investigating Causes of Low Milk Production

Rocio's Story

I suspected I had a milk supply problem at my daughter Sofia's first checkup when she hadn't gained enough. She nursed around the clock and never seemed satisfied. My first intervention was pumping after feedings to empty my breasts. I also took fenugreek and oatmeal daily for a month but saw no change, getting just 1 ounce (30 milliliters) total. Next I added a tea, and then I tried metoclopramide for a week. At two months, a lactation consultant recommended I talk to my doctor about metformin because I had PCOS (polycystic ovary syndrome). Working up to 1,500 milligrams of metformin, my supply increased to 1.5 ounces (45 milliliters) of pumped milk. Determined for more, I added 80 milligrams of domperidone and increased to 3.5 ounces (105 milliliters) per session. But despite all this milk, Sofia wasn't getting it all; after nursing she was still hungry but leaving milk in my breasts.

At six months, we finally discovered that Sofia's tight frenulum was the reason she couldn't remove milk well and I struggled so much. Minor surgery to release her frenulum was a success; my sore nipple problem resolved, and she started emptying my breasts better. I stopped the metformin and then the domperidone, maintaining my supply with just More Milk Special Blend tincture. When Sofia turned one, I finally stopped pumping and just nursed. I recall many difficult times, including when well-meaning friends and relatives would suggest I "give up." It was hard to persevere when I was tired from waking at 3:00 A.M. to pump so I could keep my supply stable or when Sofia went on a two-day nursing strike after her surgery, but with my husband's support, we made it.

CHAPTER 6

Is It Something You're Doing?

In the next five chapters, we will explore various reasons for low milk production. This is an exciting part of the journey because finding answers provides an explanation for what is happening and allows the possibility of targeting specific changes to the true cause so you can make the most milk possible.

Finding Causes of Low Milk Production

An important question to ask yourself as you begin this process is, "Was there ever a time that I felt like I had a lot of milk?" If your milk came in well but then something happened to sabotage your supply, there's a good chance that your problem will be found among the secondary causes in this chapter or the next. If your milk production seemed low from the beginning, however, or dropped off despite you and baby doing everything right, Chapters 8 through 10 about problems originating with your body may hold your answers. There may also be more than one cause. If there is both a secondary *and* primary cause, the impact upon your milk production may be even greater than if there is only one factor. For this reason, it is important to keep an open mind as you read through these possibilities because there may be unexpected answers.

The Milk Supply Equation

Sufficient glandular tissue

+ Intact nerve pathways *and* intact ducts

+ Adequate hormones *and* hormone receptors

+ **Adequately frequent, effective milk removal and stimulation (mother's side: management)**

= GOOD MILK PRODUCTION

Secondary problems can be divided into "management" and "infant" issues. Fortunately, low milk supply caused by these problems is usually reversible. The *management* problems described in this chapter are aspects of lactation that are under your control, such as how often and long you feed your baby, how you bring baby to your breast, and the possible effects of foods, herbs, and medications on your milk supply. So they may be relatively easy to fix. *Infant* problems as described in the next chapter, on the other hand, occur despite good breastfeeding management because something isn't working on baby's side of the equation.

Latch Problems

One of the most common causes of low milk production in the early weeks is poor attachment to the breast. When baby is latched too shallowly, he doesn't have enough breast in his mouth to effectively draw out milk. Less milk is removed, and the breast responds by cutting back on production.

Clues for poor attachment are usually obvious. The breasts will not soften much during nursing because milk is not being drained. Friction to the nipple causes pain and damage (*never* normal!). As the situation worsens, baby becomes fussy at breast, pulling off or falling asleep too quickly. Diaper output is scant, weight gain is inadequate, and if baby is jaundiced, the condition does not improve after the milk comes in. While initially the breasts were fuller at feeding time, they begin to feel soft and empty *all* the time.

Some well-intentioned but misinformed health care providers recommend limiting how long baby breastfeeds on each side to prevent or treat sore nipples. However, it's not how much time a baby spends at breast that causes pain but the quality of the latch and suck. Limiting the amount of time baby nurses without correcting the underlying problem can reduce milk production by limiting milk removal. A much better strategy is to determine why breastfeeding is painful in the first place and fix the problem.

The good news for latch-related supply problems is that correcting the problem is often relatively easy. See our website at www.lowmilksupply.org/latch for pointers. If you aren't able to fix it on your own, the problem could be related to baby's ability to suck effectively (see Chapter 7) and may require the help of a lactation consultant.

When Milk Seems to Dry Up Overnight

Between two and four months postpartum, some mothers experience what seems like a sudden drop in milk production. Their babies act hungry all the time, while the mothers' breasts feel empty. One possible explanation is that baby's appetite has temporarily increased due to a growth spurt. This isn't a problem unless you start giving supplemental bottles, which reduce milk removal and slow production. The result can be a downward spiral of more fussiness, more bottles, and less milk, until one day you feel like you've "just dried up."

A similar "drying up" phenomenon is related to feeding schedules that call for baby to feed every so many hours (often three or longer) by the clock. Everything seems to be working until one day the milk seems to start disappearing. The most likely explanation is inadequate development of prolactin receptors due to chronic infrequent feeding; once prolactin levels have dropped, the existing receptors cannot sustain the earlier production level. Milk supply may rebound with renewed stimulation, but other times it is difficult to resurrect. Feeding more often, possibly coupled with the addition of a galactogogue (see Chapter 12), is usually the best strategy for turning things around.

In very rare cases, this occurs despite frequent and effective feedings, due to either hormonal changes or underlying difficulties with prolactin receptors. Have a lactation consultant review your history and the clues you've collected after reading this book. The next step is to make an appointment with your physician, provide a summary of what you do right and what you've ruled out, and request hormone testing (see Chapter 9).

Stealthy Saboteurs: Common Substances That Inhibit Milk Production

In the same way that a galactogogue stimulates milk production, an *anti-galactogogue* is a substance that decreases milk production. Once you've identified and removed the offending item, milk production will often improve on its own.

Medications

Several medications are known to inhibit milk production. Bromocriptine (Parlodel), once used to dry up the milk of mothers who didn't want to breastfeed, is still used to treat excessive prolactin levels. Cabergoline (Dostinex), another prolactin inhibitor, is used more commonly because it's much safer, but its effects are longer lasting than bromocriptine. Buproprion, marketed as Wellbutrin and Zyban, has negatively affected some women's supplies. Pseudoephedrine, found in Sudafed (not Sudafed PE) and many allergy and cold medications, can also be a problem, especially in later lactation.[1] Ergot alkaloids such as methylergonovine maleate (Methergine, discussed in Chapter 9) and dopamine receptor agonists can also lower milk production.

Alcohol

The effects of alcohol (ethanol) on breastfeeding have been widely debated. Mothers have long been advised to drink a glass of beer or wine to relax and get their milk flowing. Beer especially has been recommended, and a positive effect on milk supply has indeed been documented. However, it's actually the polysaccharide from barley that stimulates milk synthesis; a good nonalcoholic beer has the same effect. Alcohol itself inhibits both the milk ejection reflex and milk production, especially when taken in large amounts. Even a moderate amount, such as a single beer or glass of wine, can disrupt the balance of lactation hormones in breastfeeding women. While the immediate effects of alcohol on milk production and delivery last only as long as the alcohol is in your system, chronic alcohol use has the potential to lower your milk supply overall.[2]

Cigarettes

Cigarettes contain nicotine, which is believed to inhibit prolactin secretion and milk production. In a classic study of both smoking and nonsmoking mothers pumping milk for their premature babies, the nonsmoking mothers were producing 25 percent more milk two weeks after birth than the mothers who smoked. At four weeks, the smoking mothers' milk supplies still were unchanged, while nonsmoking mothers increased another 20 percent. Of further concern, the fat content of the milk from smoking mothers was almost 20 percent less than that of nonsmoking mothers.[3]

Herbs

Just as there are herbs that may help increase milk production, others seem to decrease it. A lactation consultant once visited a mother whose milk came in with each baby but disappeared soon after. She watched as the mother was served a steaming bowl of homemade chicken soup heavily spiced with sage, an herb known to reduce milk supply. The mother proudly shared that her helpful husband made it for her after the birth of each baby! Once she stopped eating the soup, she was able to breastfeed exclusively for the first time. Parsley is another seasoning herb considered to have lactation-suppressing properties in large amounts, such as in a dish like tabouleh.

Peppermint is also reputed to decrease production when consumed in larger or concentrated amounts and has been used to help control some cases of oversupply. Frequent brushing with toothpaste containing real mint oil or even eating potent mint candies has caused trouble for some mothers. Jan Barger, RN, IBCLC, tells the story of a mother who called around Christmas complaining that her milk production had abruptly plummeted. It turned out that she had been eating peppermint candy canes "right and left," and once she stopped, her supply rebounded. Most of these herbs don't usually cause problems unless they are consumed regularly or in large amounts. The occasional breath mint, candy cane, or modest serving of Thanksgiving turkey stuffing seasoned with sage should not be a problem.

Hormonal Medications

Certain hormones such as estrogen, progesterone, and testosterone can inhibit milk production if their levels are too high or if synthetic versions are introduced at the wrong time during lactation. It has long been recognized that "combination" birth control pills containing forms of both estrogen and progesterone can significantly decrease milk production. Newer "minipills" are estrogen-free and better for nursing mothers, but a small number of women still experience a drop in supply until the medication is stopped. Similar problems have happened with patch and subdermal implant birth control, and a case of low supply related to a hormonal intrauterine device (IUD) has been reported. Depo-Provera, a long-acting injectable type of hormonal birth control, poses more serious problems because it lasts for three months and cannot be reversed; the best option is to try a galactogogue to counter the effect (see Chapter 12).

Hormonal birth control has a greater chance of causing problems in the early days after birth, when progesterone and estrogen receptors are plentiful, than it does later after they naturally decline post-pregnancy, reducing the effect of the hormone. Many physicians feel that a safe time to introduce these methods is around the time of your six-week postpartum checkup. However, waiting three months or longer further reduces the risk of problems.

Pregnancy

If your production has mysteriously dropped off, especially if your nipples are also newly tender, a new pregnancy might possibly be the culprit. As your body prepares for the new baby, hormones switch gears and lactation is no longer first priority. Most women begin to notice a decrease in milk production within the first several weeks; many babies also notice a difference, as both volume and taste change.

Fortunately, continuing to nurse during pregnancy will not endanger the new baby. In fact, many mothers have successfully breastfed through a pregnancy without incident. One factor that does need to be considered is the age of the current nursling when a new baby is conceived, because 70 percent of women experience a decrease in milk production by midpregnancy.[4] If the nursling is still quite young, supplementation may be necessary.

What are your options for increasing production during pregnancy? It really is a case of swimming upstream against nature, because your body shifts priority to preparing for the new baby. Nursing more often may help, but many mothers can't tolerate it because of nipple tenderness. Herbal galactogogues are another option but must be chosen carefully as some can induce contractions or have other properties of concern during pregnancy.

The dairy industry has learned that a dry period toward the end of pregnancy helps maximize milk production after the calf is born. Cows with high production in late pregnancy tend to have less milk for the new calf. So might stimulating a higher milk supply during pregnancy cause problems for the next baby's milk supply? While this question hasn't been extensively explored, human lactation expert Dr. Peter Hartmann suggests that concerned mothers consider feeding their current nursling from only one breast starting in the third trimester so that the other returns to pure colostrum production. This is a compromise between continuing to nurse the older baby and maximizing milk production after delivery.[5] While many mothers successfully use both breasts throughout pregnancy, those who barely meet baby's needs may benefit from this suggestion.

Outside Interferences

Some nursing mothers sail smoothly along until poor advice rocks their boat. This happens when a mother facing a medical procedure, drugs, or hospitalization is told that she can't nurse for a period of time, usually by staff unfamiliar with current information. To make matters worse, little or no guidance is provided on how to maintain production, and by the time breastfeeding is "allowed" again, milk supply is damaged. Educating yourself on the facts is your best defense, and regular pumping your backup. Consider if the person telling you that you can't breastfeed is up to date on lactation information. *Always get a second opinion from someone with expertise and resources in lactation before following advice to stop breastfeeding.* Dr. Thomas Hale's book, *Medications and Mothers' Milk* (updated biannually) is an excellent safety reference. You or the person questioning breastfeeding can then discuss this information with baby's health care provider.

Feeding Frequency and Duration

Newborns must feed frequently to fuel their growth and get your milk production up and running. Your job is to make sure that baby has all the opportunities he needs. The following can interfere with this process and sabotage your milk factory if they aren't caught early.

The Sleepy or Nondemanding Baby

There is an old saying, "Let sleeping dogs and babies lie." Sounds like a good idea, especially if you've been told to feed the baby "on cue" and he isn't "asking" at the moment, right? While this advice is fine for an older baby who is gaining well, it isn't appropriate for a newborn who is jaundiced, lethargic, or not gaining weight well.

Excessive sleepiness has several possible causes. A newborn may be drowsy after delivery because of medications given to you during labor. The effects may be brief, or they can linger for several days. During this time, lots of skin-to-skin contact can help stimulate your baby and trigger his nursing instincts.

Simply not getting enough milk can also cause a baby to sleep too much. He may eventually rouse and show clear signs of hunger but fall asleep again within minutes at the breast if the milk isn't flowing quickly or he doesn't have much energy to feed. This in turn leads to needing longer periods of sleep to conserve precious energy. Until milk production can be increased, this baby needs supplementation for energy to feed well at breast. Becoming fatigued during a feeding and falling asleep too soon can also happen as a result of suck or medical problems on baby's side (discussed in Chapter 7).

Another cause of infant drowsiness is *jaundice*, a temporary yellowing of the skin that often looks like a suntan. Normal *physiologic* jaundice is caused by elevated levels of a blood by-product called *bilirubin* and is a healthy response to moving to life outside the womb. Early and frequent feedings minimize jaundice by stimulating bowel movements, through which bilirubin is eliminated. Water isn't helpful because it produces only urine. If bilirubin levels rise significantly in the early days, enticing baby to eat is more challenging because bilirubin makes babies sleepy and lethargic. *While babies need to eat to get rid of the bilirubin, sleepy babies can be difficult to feed.* A jaundiced baby should be awakened to feed at least every two to three hours until he begins to wake more on his own. Gentle methods such as holding him upright, massaging his body, talking to him, undressing him, or changing his diaper are most likely to result in willingness to feed.

Babies usually need more of mother's milk, not less, to resolve jaundice. But a baby whose bilirubin levels are very high and unresponsive to regular management may require temporary suspension of breastfeeding (usually twenty-four to forty-eight hours) and feedings of an elemental formula until levels begin to drop.[6] It is critical to maintain frequent, thorough milk removal by other methods until baby can do the job himself again.

Pacifiers

Pacifiers can mask the hunger cues of babies who are easily soothed by them. They are often given in the belief that baby is supposed to be full after so many minutes at breast and stay content for a certain amount of time. An assertive baby will spit it out and insist on more milk, but an easygoing baby may not be as persistent. This can disrupt the baby-driven milk-making process by forcing inappropriately long feeding intervals that ultimately reduce milk supply. Pacifiers may also affect baby's suck, further decreasing the amount of milk made. Although the American Academy of Pediatrics work group on sudden infant death syndrome (SIDS) recommended pacifiers in 2006, forgoing them in order to protect your milk supply does not increase the risk of SIDS when your baby is allowed to nurse whenever and wherever he desires.[7]

Busyness

Juggling a baby and the conflicting demands of a busy household is challenging. Feedings can be unconsciously postponed when you're preoccupied by other tasks, trying to get "just one more thing" done. It's especially difficult if you have older children and are always on the run driving them around, and the temptation to put off feedings instead of taking time to nurse right now may be strong.

In the midst of all that you have to do, it may be hard to remember how long you used to spend sitting and feeding your first children, but think back carefully. Are there differences that might be contributing to the problem you're experiencing now? Though this may sound difficult, it is crucial to slow down and remember that *this* baby will only be young once, and his needs are immediate and important. Keeping him close in a soft baby carrier can help you respond to early feeding cues while on the go.

Clock-Driven Feeding Durations and Feeding Schedules

When do you eat supper? How long does it take? Is it always the same time of day, and do you always take the same amount of time? Probably not. Yet, it's common for mothers to be told that they should nurse only every so many hours or for a certain number of minutes on each side.

Traditional cultures understand that babies should be put to the breast when they ask and nursed as long as they wish, and that how often and how long varies according to each baby's emotional and physical needs at any given time. In our society, however, we tend to believe that babies should breastfeed only for nutrition. Mothers are urged to get baby on a schedule as quickly as possible to instill early discipline, to fit him conveniently into family life, to make life more predictable, or for "sleep training." Whatever a parent's fear or motivation, schedules are often regarded as an important parenting goal.

Some authors claim that babies who are fed when they want will never learn delayed gratification.[8] Schedules are touted as essential for parental survival and are sometimes promoted under the premise that "teaching" babies to self-soothe and be independent is necessary for healthy development. But the opposite is true: studies show that babies whose parents respond to their cues for feeding and comfort cry less and are more confident and secure as they grow up.[9]

Schedules may seem helpful to parents, but they don't always meet the needs of breastfeeding mothers and babies. Rather than allowing milk production to be driven by baby as nature designed, schedules artificially determine when feedings will take place. Mothers with abundant production and vigorously nursing babies may do well, but mothers with marginal supplies or babies with difficulties often do not. Even if all looks well in the beginning, a sudden drop-off in production can happen after a few months if an insufficient number of hormone receptors were established in the early weeks.[10]

Some books now tout "flexible routines" as a more reasonable approach to feeding baby. While they are an improvement, the "flexibility" in these new methods translates to bending only on

81

special occasions such as growth spurts, with the goal of getting back to the designated schedule as soon as possible. Bottom line: advice that supersedes your instincts on when to feed your baby can undermine your milk supply.

Your Need for Sleep

New mothers can become obsessed with sleep simply because it's hard to get enough. Sleep deprivation can drive us to desperation, and the around-the-clock needs of young babies can seem like an impossible demand to meet. Mothers in traditional cultures tend to take babies' nighttime needs in stride, but Western living involves clocks, deadlines, schedules, and appointments that don't always suit a baby's way of life. Is it any wonder that we feel stressed over lack of sleep and fear that this stage of life will never end?

The desire for more sleep is the most common reason given for nighttime bottles. But each skipped feeding decreases milk production by that same amount unless you compensate by pumping, preferably at about the same time, which defeats the purpose of a relief bottle. Realistic expectations are important. If your newborn feeds eight to twelve times a day and you want him to sleep eight hours at night so that you can have a long stretch of uninterrupted sleep, when is he going to get those feedings in? He has just sixteen hours, which means he needs to nurse every two hours, assuming adequate breast storage capacity and that baby isn't taking milk faster than it is being made after a long night of inactivity. Can you really accommodate this? It is more realistic and normal for a baby to space his feedings throughout the day and night.

It's easier to breastfeed at night if baby is in bed with you or sleeping nearby. You may not even wake up completely while baby nurses. Co-sleeping is a time-honored tradition that has unfortunately come under fire as newspaper headlines inflame parents' fears of overlying. However, Dr. James McKenna and other infant sleep researchers have shown conclusively that babies and mothers are biologically hardwired to sleep together, affording them not only more rest but safer sleep for babies. If you choose to co-sleep, be sure to do so in a safe manner, just as it's important that a crib be used in a safe manner. For more information, read Dr. McKenna's book, *Sleeping with Your Baby: A Parent's Guide to Cosleeping*, and visit the Kellymom website at www.kellymom.com/parenting/sleep/familybed.html.

Unnecessary Supplementation

There are certainly times when baby isn't getting enough milk and must be supplemented. But there are also times when unnecessary supplements sabotage milk production by reducing milk removal and stretching out feeding intervals. The Santa Barbara County Breastfeeding Coalition studied reasons mothers stopped breastfeeding before baby was a year old and found that mothers often introduced bottles *before* problems with milk production developed, rarely noticing a connection to their eventual loss of milk supply. Problems usually start with "just one bottle a day" or "just a few bottles a week," but the more supplements given, the more are needed because milk isn't made when it isn't removed. It becomes a slippery slope where bottle-feeding eventually seems more convenient or baby appears to like it better. Gratuitous supplementation is the sneakiest cause of management-induced low milk production because it "just sort of happens."

Are Bottles Really Necessary?

Even when regular separations aren't planned, bottles are often introduced out of concern that baby won't accept them later on. This is realistic in that there does seem to be a window of opportunity in the first three months when babies are more willing to take a bottle. But if you won't be away from baby on a regular basis, there's really no need to introduce one. In an emergency, he could be fed by cup, spoon, or other devices and will survive. Introducing a bottle just so baby will take one for an unplanned future event isn't necessary and may undermine your milk supply. It makes more sense for bottle-feeding mothers to make sure their babies can breastfeed . . . just in case no formula is available!

Another reason frequently given to use bottles is for others to bond with baby. This is one of society's great myths. The truth is that *baby bonds to those who hold, touch, and love him, not just the person who feeds him.* Do you feed your partner in order to bond, or is touch the magic ingredient? Helping family members to find other ways—such as burping, baths, and massages—to connect with baby is a much better alternative than having them compete with you for feeding opportunities. Even if you're pumping milk for the bottle, this can interrupt the early mother-baby dance and lead to baby preferring the bottle, especially if there have been any difficulties with breastfeeding.

Nutrition

Mothers often worry that they aren't eating enough of the "right" foods to maintain adequate milk production. Yet most mothers will produce enough milk even when their eating habits aren't the best. And if caloric intake is low, a nursing mother's prolactin levels rise, apparently to compensate. It's only when you're *severely* malnourished that the quantity or quality of your milk can diminish significantly. Most of the time, your own body will suffer before baby does.[11] However, there *are* certain foods reputed to promote good milk production that may be helpful to some mothers (see Chapter 12).

Gradual weight loss through moderate dieting will not reduce your milk production. However, a sudden, dramatic decrease in calories over several days or longer (such as crash dieting) can lower it by forcing the body to cut back on noncritical uses of energy to ensure its own threatened survival. Consuming at least 1,500 to 1,800 calories per day is the minimum amount most women need to maintain their supply.[12]

Eating Disorders

Mothers with a history of eating disorders such as anorexia or bulimia can usually breastfeed fully, especially if body weight is back to normal. Milk production during active eating disorders has not been studied, but it seems reasonable to assume that loss of fat reserves and "starving" the body can force it into survival mode, resulting in decreased milk output. Milk composition may also be affected, although this has not yet been studied. It is known that some bulimic women do not experience the full nighttime surge of prolactin and that the effect is tied to the frequency of bingeing. If you're struggling with an eating disorder while breastfeeding, consider consulting a nutritionist, who can help you maximize your nutritional intake.[13]

Mothers who follow a vegetarian or vegan diet may be at risk for insufficient amounts of B_{12}, which may cause a loss of appetite and drowsiness in a breastfeeding baby, with a corresponding decrease in milk production.[14] For this reason, vitamin B_{12} is recommended for breastfeeding mothers who follow a strict vegetarian or vegan diet.

Gastric Bypass Surgery

With the rise in surgical treatments for obesity, breastfeeding after gastric bypass surgery is a hot new topic. Cases of low milk production have been reported by lactation consultants even though the medical literature currently reflects only problems with B_{12} deficiency in some patients' milk. Women who have the Roux-en-Y procedure especially are at risk for calcium, folate, vitamin B_{12}, iron, and protein deficiencies.[15] One mother experienced significant problems with milk production until she discovered that her zinc was low and her B_{12} was "very low-normal." When she began taking supplements of both nutrients, her milk production increased to normal levels. Blood tests will show if you are absorbing enough nutrients.

Women who have gastric bypass surgery are often encouraged by their doctors to avoid pregnancy in the first two years after surgery while they are healing and completing their most rapid period of weight loss. During that time they are mostly metabolizing fat, and their low caloric intake makes it difficult to consume enough essential nutrients to adequately support pregnancy and lactation.[16] Once they pass this period, gastric bypass mothers who consume at least seventy grams of protein per day along with vitamin supplements generally don't have trouble making milk.[17] But it is also important to consider that low milk production after bypass surgery may be related to preexisting hormonal conditions associated with obesity (discussed in Chapter 9).

Hydration

A pervasive myth in many cultures is that not drinking enough water causes low milk supply. While it's true that life-threatening, *severe* dehydration may cause your body to cut back on milk production, the mild dehydration that most of us operate under does not. An old but still valid study from 1939 reported that nursing mothers who were given one liter less of water a day than was recommended continued to produce plenty of milk.[18]

The flip side of this belief is that drinking more water makes more milk, which is just as wrong; in fact, drinking too much water can actually *decrease* milk production rather than increase it. The body's reaction to excessive water intake (well beyond thirst) is to dump the excess fluid through the urine in order to maintain the proper electrolyte balance.[19] Water is diverted away from the breast, and lower milk volume can result. Dr. Christina Smillie explains the misconception this way: Milk production doesn't increase because of drinking more fluid; it is actually the other way around. Women who make lots of milk will be thirsty in order to replace the fluid they use to produce milk. When a mother is making less milk, she does not need to drink as much. Until an increased demand stimulates higher supply, the excess forced fluids will be wasted, and you'll just urinate more. The best advice is to *drink to thirst*. Keep your urine a pale yellow, and you'll be drinking just the right amount to make milk.

CHAPTER 7

Is It Something Your Baby Is Doing?

Now that you've considered the factors under your control that can affect milk production, it's time to explore those that affect baby's ability to nurse effectively. If your milk production decreased because your baby has been unable to remove milk well, it can be a challenge to narrow the possible reasons down to an actual cause. You may need to work closely with your pediatrician and lactation consultant to find definite answers. The information in this chapter will help by providing an overview of reasons babies may not be able to breastfeed effectively.

The Milk Supply Equation

Sufficient glandular tissue
+ Intact nerve pathways *and* ducts
+ Adequate hormones *and* hormone receptors
+ **Adequately frequent, effective milk removal and stimulation (baby's side)**

= GOOD MILK PRODUCTION

Suck Problems

Effective sucking depends on baby's ability to coordinate the use of his tongue, cheeks, palate, jaw, facial muscles, and lips. Any significant variations or problems may affect his ability to remove milk efficiently.

The clearest evidence for a sucking problem is painful nursing and a nipple that comes out of baby's mouth significantly misshapen, bruised, cracked, or bleeding. On the other hand, a baby with a weak suck isn't able to draw out his mother's nipple much at all. As mentioned in Chapter 5, the longer a mother receives pain medications during labor, the greater the chance they will affect baby's sucking ability until his body has eliminated them. Suck problems can also occur as the result of anatomical malformations or underlying problems such as torticollis, a tightening of some of the neck muscles. Newborns can develop disorganized sucking habits as a result of not getting enough milk out of the breast: they were born sucking well, but then their sucking movements deteriorated as they desperately tried alternate ways to get milk from the breast. Babies are smart, and when one thing doesn't work, they try another. Once they experience a little success at the breast and discover the movements that draw milk out most effectively, the suck often improves spontaneously without any other intervention.

Accurately identifying and resolving suck problems can be a challenge even for lactation consultants. The first steps are to ensure that baby is latching as deeply as possible, feed him adequately in a way that is supportive of breastfeeding while you work to solve the problem, and pump as needed to maintain maximum milk production. When those bases are covered, some lactation consultants may refer you to another specialist for suck training exercises or special feeding methods that encourage baby to move his tongue more effectively. At-breast supplementers or special bottle nipples may also be used. If these techniques don't work, baby should be evaluated by a healthcare provider who specializes in identifying and treating suck dysfunction.

When anatomical problems have been thoroughly assessed and ruled out, therapies that treat nerve impingements or other subtle interferences are worth exploring. Some babies respond positively to infant oral motor function therapy by a speech or occupational therapist.[1] Chiropractic treatment also can be effective in improving some suck problems.[2] A third option is craniosacral therapy (CST), a very gentle manipulation of the plates of the skull to release subtle pressures on nerves affecting muscles and reflexes. CST has been effective in improving some suck problems.[3]

Tongue-Tie

A baby's ability to draw milk from the breast depends on his ability to move his tongue freely. In order to grasp an adequate amount of breast for latching deeply, his tongue must *comfortably* extend past his lower lip. To stabilize the breast, the sides of the tongue need to be able cup it. Finally, the tip of the tongue needs to be able to lift higher than halfway when the mouth is open, while the back of the tongue needs to lift and then drop to create the vacuum that pulls out milk. Infants with tongue-tie, also known as *ankyloglossia*, lack the tongue mobility to breastfeed effectively because the membrane that connects the base of the tongue to the floor of the mouth, called the *lingual frenulum* or *frenum*, is too tight and restrictive. While a normal frenulum is hard to see in an infant, a tight frenulum attaches on the bottom side of the tongue anywhere from the base of the tongue to the tip and connects to the floor of the mouth anywhere from the base of the tongue to the top of baby's gum ridge. It may look like a thin, stretchy web that is almost transparent, or it may be more like a thick rope or knot. A submucosal frenulum runs under the floor of the mouth, often pulling the floor up when baby tries to lift his tongue, like a rope pulling up the center of a carpet. Any type of tight frenulum can lead to feeding fatigue, poor milk transfer, slow weight gain, and ultimately, low milk production if the baby cannot remove milk effectively from the breast.[4]

Because tongue-ties occur in a number of variations, the effect on baby's suck depends on where the frenulum connects. With an attachment close to or at the front of the tongue, only the sides of the tongue can rise when baby tries to lift it, sometimes forming a characteristic heart shape. A notch may be visible at the tip when he attempts to extend his tongue, or the tongue tip may even roll downward. When the frenulum is attached tightly at the base of the tongue, the tip is able to lift more but still not as much as it should, while the back cannot rise and drop enough to create a good vacuum. As a result, a frenulum attached too tightly to the base of the tongue can be even more problematic.[5]

Clues that a baby is tongue-tied include latch trouble, sucking blisters on the lips, chronic sore nipples, "clicking" or "popping" sounds during breastfeeding, a persistently abraded nipple, or a flattened nipple when baby unlatches. A "bunching" of the back of the tongue may be felt as baby tries unsuccessfully to maneuver, resulting in friction to the nipple. He may have difficulty opening his mouth widely enough to latch deeply because the tight frenulum is pulling on the hyoid bone in the neck that supports the root of the tongue, which in turn pulls the jaw muscles. Inadequate feedings are common as baby wears out from his efforts before his tummy is full, and tongue tremors may be visible as he tires. He may fall asleep quickly and awaken hungrily a little later, or feedings may feel more like marathons as he slowly keeps working to fill his belly.

The most common treatment, *frenotomy*, divides the membrane with surgical scissors or laser to release the tongue. In most cases, a frenulum connected to the front part of the tongue is very thin with little or no blood vessels or nerves in it, so there is very little bleeding or discomfort when it's cut. A tight frenulum at the base of the tongue is thicker and so may bleed slightly more. The procedure itself takes only seconds; baby may feel some stinging, but generally a frenotomy is no more traumatic than an immunization shot, and in most cases baby can usually be put to the breast within a minute or so for soothing. Frenotomy is safe, rarely has complications, and is highly effective when performed correctly.[6]

After the procedure, your lactation consultant may suggest special exercises to help baby relearn effective tongue movements. Until the frenotomy can be done, or especially if it isn't done for some reason, it may be necessary to pump after feedings to ensure thorough milk removal and provide any necessary supplement.

Lactation consultants usually know local health care providers—often ear, nose, and throat (ENT) specialists—who are able to knowledgeably assess and treat a tight frenulum. Some less experienced providers will acknowledge the impact of tongue-tie on breastfeeding but suggest waiting to see if the frenulum will stretch or break on its own. This may not happen enough or at all, though, which is why there are older people who still have a tight frenulum. Rather, the mouth will enlarge as baby grows so that he is able to take in more breast tissue; it is hoped this would improve stabilization and milk transfer, but it does not always do so. Relying on this enlargement is likely to jeopardize your milk supply and decrease the likelihood of successful breastfeeding.

If weaning is recommended, this eliminates only the breastfeeding issue. Babies with a tight frenulum can still have difficulty with bottle-feeding, speech impediments, reflux, dental malformations (eventually requiring orthodontic care), indigestion, snoring, and sleep apnea. Tight frenulums can even make swallowing pills and licking ice cream cones difficult.[7]

While tongue-tie is the most well-known type of frenulum restriction, another type that can also cause latch problems involves a similar membrane inside the center of the upper and lower lips, called the *labial frenum* or *frenulum*. When this membrane is tight, it may prevent baby from flanging his lips widely, and he may purse them instead, resulting in a shallower latch. If it extends into the upper gum, it can cause a gap between the front teeth that becomes more prominent in adulthood. Labial frenulum restrictions can occur alone or together with tongue-tie and are also easily treated during infancy.

In discussing the possibility of tongue-tie with your baby's doctor, it may be helpful to refer him or her to *Supporting Sucking Skills in Breastfeeding Infants* by Catherine Watson Genna, B.S., IBCLC,

The Murphy Maneuver

If baby is having trouble breastfeeding and you aren't sure if he is tongue-tied, San Diego pediatrician Dr. James Murphy suggests pushing your little finger to the base of the tongue on one side and sweeping it across to the other side to see what you can feel. If you feel little or no resistance more than a small "speed bump," then most likely there is no problem. Should you feel a large speed bump that you can get past with a little more effort, it is most likely a "tree trunk" frenulum, a short, wide band of tissue buried in the floor of the mouth and attached to the base of the tongue. It usually, though not always, restricts tongue movements and causes latch problems even though it *looks* like there isn't enough there to be a problem. When you can't sweep your finger across without pulling it back to "jump over a fence," the frenulum is a fibrous band attached closer to the front of the tongue. It may be buried underneath the floor of the mouth or visible as an external web. If you see a narrow white streak running down the middle of the floor of the mouth that feels like a wire, it usually extends to the front of the tongue like a string. Pushing your finger into this "piano wire" frenulum will often cause the tip of the tongue to tilt downward and the center of the tongue to pull down and crease along the middle. "Tree trunk," "fence," and "piano wire" frenulums are red flags for significant tongue function impairment.

for detailed tongue-tie diagnostic criteria and treatment information. If your baby's doctor is reluctant to treat the frenulum but you believe that treatment would benefit you and baby, don't hesitate to ask your lactation consultant for a referral to another practitioner who is familiar with their diagnosis and treatment. We also maintain a listing at www.lowmilksupply.org/frenotomy.shtml.

Palatal Variations

Variations in the shape of the palate may affect baby's ability to maintain the suction that helps keep the breast in his mouth and creates the vacuum to remove milk. You can feel your baby's palate by offering him a clean finger to suck on, with the pad of your finger pointing up. A normal hard palate slopes gently upward from front to back until it becomes the soft palate in the back. The sides are wide, and the pad of your finger should rest comfortably in it, touching the top.

High Palate

A high palate is shaped like a dome with steep sides, and the top is not as easily touched when baby sucks on your finger (pad side up). Variations that feel like a fingerprint indentation are known as "bubble" palates. Babies who have high palates may not be comfortable drawing the breast in deeply and tend to gag easily. After initially latching deeply, they often pull back into a shallower position where suction breaks more easily, frequently causing characteristic clicking sounds.

While some unusual variations in palate shape can be genetic, most high palates are caused by problems with tongue mobility.[8] As the baby grows in the womb, the tongue shapes and spreads the palate. When tongue movement is restricted, so is spreading. Bubble palates and tongue-tie are commonly found together.

A baby with a high palate needs to be encouraged to accept the breast more deeply in his mouth. Lying on your back with baby on top of you, tummy to tummy, can help by naturally encouraging head extension and drawing the hyoid bone forward to increase baby's tongue reach and grasp. Whatever position you nurse in, encourage him to open his mouth widely and keep him tucked close to the breast. CST and treatment for tongue-tie, if present, can be effective in helping the palate to spread after birth. In the meantime, extra pumping may be needed to maintain your milk supply.

Cleft Palate

Probably the best-known palatal problem is a *cleft of the hard palate*, with or without cleft lip. When there is an opening in the hard palate, it's almost impossible for baby to create the vacuum necessary to hold the breast and draw out milk. Babies with only a cleft lip should be able to form a good seal if they are positioned in a way that allows the soft tissue of the breast to fill in the cleft. Those with a cleft of the hard palate, however, are rarely able to form an effective seal, even with an obturator (a customized device that temporarily covers the cleft).

The baby with a *cleft of the soft palate* has similar problems and challenges. Because the hole is less visible, it may not be noticed in the early newborn exams and may be detected only when baby has difficulty feeding.

A subtle, lesser-known variation is a *submucosal cleft of the soft palate*. The surface of the soft palate is intact, but there is an opening in the muscle underneath that may cause an inadequate closing of the soft palate muscle, known as the velopharyngeal sphincter, resulting in a condition called *velopharyngeal insufficiency*. This condition makes it difficult for the baby to maintain adequate suction. Submucosal clefts are hard to detect. There may be a slight V-shaped notch where the hard and soft palates meet, and the uvula, the hanging flap of tissue in the back of the mouth, may be split. A baby with a submucosal cleft will have difficulty staying attached to the breast and may slip off easily when you move. Clicking sounds from suction breaks frequently occur when he is nursing. On occasion, milk may come out of his nose as he feeds or spits up. Most tellingly, he may not gain weight well. Interventions for submucosal clefts of the soft palate are rare. Because they are tricky to identify, time may have elapsed and milk production may be diminished before the situation is discovered. If baby's suck feels weak and neither you nor your lactation consultant can pinpoint the problem, ask your pediatrician to observe a feeding and examine baby's mouth more thoroughly to rule out anatomical problems. If the pediatrician can't determine the source of the problem, ask for a referral to an ear, nose, and throat specialist, or otolaryngologist, for a more thorough evaluation.

Facial Abnormalities

Cleft lips are one form of facial abnormality. Others include non-symmetric facial features, which may become more noticeable as baby grows, or small jaws, called *micrognathia*. When the chin and lower jaw are small in relation to the rest of the face, baby's tongue is also small, making it difficult to extend it out far enough to breastfeed effectively. Some babies go on nursing strikes or eventually refuse to eat solids because it hurts to move the jaw. There may also be underlying facial nerve damage affecting suck. Special positioning and latch techniques may be required to help this baby breastfeed. In many cases, he just needs time to grow in order to breastfeed well. In the meantime, pumping will help to maintain good milk production.

Airway Problems

A baby who cannot breathe easily will have difficulty coordinating sucking and swallowing with breathing, which makes it challenging to remove milk well enough to sustain good milk production. Sometimes the cause is as simple as secretions blocking the nostrils. These can be softened with your milk or sterile saline water and then gently suctioned out prior to feeding. Chronic stuffy noses may be due to allergies, and removing the offending substances from the environment or your diet may help. Talk with baby's health care provider for guidance about minimizing allergy symptoms. Narrow nasal passages or other structural blockages of the nose can also interfere with breathing when baby is eating. Fortunately, as baby grows larger, the passages usually enlarge as well. In rare cases, surgery may be required.

Laryngomalacia and *tracheomalacia* occur when parts of the larynx, pharynx, or trachea (windpipe) are "floppy" due to poor development, causing a high, squeaky, wheezy sound known as *stridor* when

95

baby cries or feeds. Baby may struggle at the breast, feeding in very short sucking bursts (three to five sucks) with long breaks to recover. He also may hold his breath for several sucks and swallows or let go of the breast entirely in order to gasp and pant and catch his breath. He often ends the feeding before he is full simply because he is too tired to continue. As a result, he may not take in enough milk to gain weight well, and milk production may suffer over time. Severe cases are usually caught early and only rarely corrected with surgery. The more common mild to moderate cases often go unnoticed unless they are causing a problem. These conditions usually resolve on their own by the end of baby's second year.

Maintaining as open an airway as possible is crucial if your baby has breathing issues. Position him at the breast with his neck extended back to open the airway further and make breathing easier for him. Keeping him in a more upright position is also helpful. Pacing the feedings by initiating periodic breaks before he falls behind is usually necessary, especially if baby routinely holds his breath for too long. Milk production may need to be supported with pumping until feedings improve.

Cardiac Problems

Babies who have heart problems breathe more rapidly to get enough oxygen into their bodies. They tire easily in normal activities and so may end feedings before they get all the milk they need. A feeding strategy that minimizes the effort they expend is important since their faster breathing and heart rates use more calories. Breastfeeding is easier than bottle-feeding and provides higher and more stable oxygen levels.[9] Massaging the breast before feeding and breast compression during feeding can help get more milk into baby with less effort on his part. It may be necessary to pump after feedings in order to maintain an adequate supply. Many babies with cardiac difficulties do well with at-breast supplementation, but others may require supplementary bottles. The good news is that these babies usually breastfeed much better after the heart defect is corrected surgically.

Nervous System Issues

Nerves send messages to the brain about sensations such as pressure, taste, or temperature and also allow the brain to direct the actions of muscles, including those used for sucking, swallowing, and breathing. Nervous system–related feeding issues can result from hereditary problems, prenatal drug exposure (recreational or prescription), trauma, cerebral palsy, Bell's palsy, or certain other medical conditions. Some nervous system issues can be explained by developmental immaturity, while in other cases there is no good explanation at all. Whatever the cause, it may take time for baby's sucking to improve. Some babies with nervous system issues need supplementary feedings, which may require you to pump in addition to breastfeeding to maintain your milk supply.

Hypotonia

Low muscle tone, or *hypotonia*, is common in babies with Down syndrome but can also occur in other infants with neurological issues. Babies with low muscle tone have difficulty with all aspects of latching and sucking—getting a good seal on the breast, maintaining suction, and using the tongue properly to remove milk. The suck may feel weak or "light." There may be dimples in baby's cheeks while feeding, and because he does not maintain suction well, he may fall off the breast easily. Babies with low muscle tone may tense key muscles around the lips in an attempt to stabilize their position at the breast and compensate for other muscles that are not doing their job. This can be tiring and stressful. Baby may nurse well at first, but as the muscles tire, it becomes more difficult to remove milk well. Hypotonic babies tend to nurse better later in the day and into the night as they slowly gather tension in their bodies.

The Dancer hold is a special way of holding the breast while simultaneously supporting baby's face to stabilize his jaw and cheeks so that he can put all his energy into sucking. When cradling baby in your arm, slide your opposite hand under your breast, palm up, and put your thumb on one side of baby's lower jaw and your index finger on the opposite side. Curl your third finger and place lightly under baby's chin (you'll have two fingers left under the breast).

Babies with hypotonia also benefit from being flexed at the hips while nursing because it helps them organize their sucking better. Good flexion keeps ear, shoulder, and hip in line but bends baby at the hip joint so that he "wraps" or "curls" around your body.

Hypertonia

Infants with *hypertonia* have very tight, tense muscles. Their bodies feel stiff, and they don't flex, cuddle, or relax easily into a parent's arms. They tend to breastfeed fitfully and poorly, popping on and off the breast. It is not uncommon for them to clench their jaws while nursing or even clamp down on the breast with their gums. Because of the feeding difficulties, your nipples may be sore and your breasts may not get enough stimulation to sustain good milk production.

Hypertonicity can be a physical trait that is present much of the time, or it can be a behavior that expresses baby's negative feelings about a situation. When it is related to an emotional response, the baby will feel cuddly when he is not being stressed. Stiffness and arching happen only when he is put to the breast, which he may associate with previous oral trauma such as overly aggressive suctioning of the mouth at birth. Babies with true hypertonia feel stiff or tense at times unrelated to feedings.

Hypertonic infants tend to nurse best in the night and morning hours, before the day's tensions increase their muscle tone still more. Prior to breastfeeding, try placing baby in a blanket with the four corners gathered and then swing gently in a head-to-toe direction to help him relax. Rocking or walking around with baby snuggled closely, even skin to skin, may help. Swaddling baby into a moderately flexed position is another technique that may calm him and help him to focus. Positioning baby by your side with his feet pointing behind you, commonly called the "football" or "clutch" hold, to feed can help maintain this flexed position, as will holding baby in the traditional position with his chest against your abdomen and his hips flexed to wrap around your side. Conversely, some hypertonic babies breastfeed better when allowed to stretch out on a pillow. Experiment with different approaches to find what works best for your baby.

Sensory Processing Disorders

Sensory processing disorders, also known as *sensory integration dysfunction*, are not easily diagnosed in an infant. Sensations that are usually interesting or pleasant, such as the brush of a hand or a soft touch, can be aggravating and even intolerable to these infants. They are often irritable, adapt poorly to changes in their environment, and may seem terrified of movement. They find it hard to tolerate noise and the touching involved in baths or diaper changes. Or they may seem to crave movement, needing to be carried much of the time. Some have difficulty interpreting sensations and actively try to avoid those that bother them. These sensitive infants may not breastfeed well because they are overwhelmed by sensory input and will arch away from the breast, cry, latch poorly, and release the breast frequently, which can be mistaken for high or low supply.[10] Milk production can suffer over time if baby does not breastfeed effectively due to his heightened sensitivity. Sensory defensive infants often respond better to firm touch with deep pressure; smooth, soft fabrics without irritating zippers, tags, or rough seams; swaddling; swinging head to toe before breastfeeding; breastfeeding in a sling; and low light and noise levels during feeding.

Some sensory defensive infants may feel calmer with direct skin-to-skin contact rather than being clothed or swaddled. Others breastfeed better with minimal touching, sometimes preferring to rest on a pillow on your lap rather than being held in your arms. Babies who do not sense the breast well while latching may respond best when the nipple is aimed downward toward their tongue rather than toward the palate. They also may be more willing to latch on to a nipple shield because of the firm sensation it provides.

If you suspect that your baby's latch or sucking problems may be due to sensory issues, discuss your observations with your pediatrician and request a referral to an occupational therapist or early intervention program for a formal assessment. These experts are trained to help infants with sensory processing disorders and can provide helpful guidance. A skilled lactation consultant may also have ideas to help your baby nurse better and can work with the occupational therapist. The Sensory Processing Disorder Network (www.spdnetwork.org) has more resources. In the meantime, you may need to do supportive pumping until baby is able to handle the job adequately himself.

The Large, Small, or Early Baby

Gestational age and overall development at birth can affect a newborn's ability to thrive at the breast and maintain adequate milk production. Premature babies have less stamina and can fatigue quickly; they may also have poorer muscle tone that interferes with effective suckling (see Chapter 14). Borderline early babies (thirty-five to thirty-seven weeks) can look deceptively normal yet not be mature enough to nurse well. Infants who are small or large for gestational age have been affected by something in the uterine environment that may also affect their ability to breastfeed. In all of these situations, "insurance pumping" after feedings is wise until baby is breastfeeding well enough to maintain a good milk supply.

Infections

In some cases of poor infant growth, an underlying infection, such as a urinary tract infection, may be the culprit. Energy requirements may be higher and growth can slow down when the body is fighting an infection. If baby is suddenly not feeding well or his weight gain has slowed down, it is important to ask your doctor if underlying infections or other health conditions could be the cause.

Gastroesophageal Reflux Disease

All babies spit up some, and some babies spit up a lot. Most of the time it is largely a laundry problem. But there are babies who have such significant problems with milk coming back up (reflux) that eating becomes painful and unpleasant. Their condition may be obvious because they regurgitate large amounts after and in between feedings, or they may have a "silent" version of reflux in which partially digested milk comes just far enough up the esophagus to cause burning sensations and sometimes interfere with breathing, making baby cry and choke. This is usually diagnosed as *gastroesophageal reflux disease* (GERD). Infants with GERD may begin to associate feeding with negative consequences ("I eat, then I hurt") and then put off feedings, eating only when they absolutely have to, resulting in slow weight gain. This, of course, can affect milk production as well.

GERD often is simply a problem of immaturity, but it also may be triggered by sensitivity to a protein, often dairy in your diet, that passes into the milk. Sometimes it can even be a mechanical issue such as misalignment of the spine or cranial plates, or a side effect of tongue-tie. Regardless of the cause, all babies with GERD benefit from smaller, more frequent meals; having their heads higher than their bottoms during feedings; being kept upright for twenty minutes after eating; and being laid down to rest with the head of the bed elevated. Medication may be prescribed, and sometimes tests are necessary to determine exactly what is happening. If your production is low because baby doesn't seem to like breastfeeding and exhibits some of these behaviors, it may be helpful to discuss the possibility of GERD with his doctor. In the meantime, if necessary, you know what to do to maintain your milk production—pump! That will buy you time until breastfeeding improves.

CHAPTER 8

Is It Something About Your Breasts?

Of all the causes of low milk production, those due to an inherent primary problem with your breasts or physiology can be the most mysterious and frustrating. It may be difficult to tell if the root issue is temporary or long-term. Those that are short-term usually resolve on their own so long as breastfeeding continues to be managed well. Long-term primary problems result from either anatomical causes, such as breast structure problems, or physiological causes, which are often related to genetic or hormonal dysfunctions. This chapter delves into the known anatomical factors that can affect milk production, while Chapter 9 discusses physiological factors. If nothing you've read so far seems to fit, these chapters may shed more light on your situation.

The Milk Supply Equation

   Sufficient glandular tissue

+ **Intact nerve pathways and ducts**

+ Adequate hormones *and* hormone receptors

+ Adequately frequent, effective milk removal and stimulation

= GOOD MILK PRODUCTION

Do you have any of the following risk factors for anatomical problems?

☐ Breast or chest surgery or medical procedures, even as an infant

☐ Injury to your chest during childhood or adolescence

☐ Damage to any nerves or a spinal cord injury

☐ Unusual breast or nipple features, such as one breast being much smaller than the other or a nipple that's divided into two sections

☐ Little or no breast tenderness or changes during pregnancy or after birth

☐ A chronic illness or condition

Anatomical Variations

Nature doesn't always form every part of our bodies perfectly. Anatomical variations also can result from accident, disease, ill-

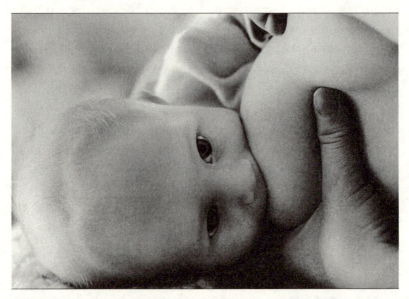

Making a "breast sandwich" can help some babies to latch, stay on, and get more milk.

ness, or surgery. Whatever the cause, structural problems with your milk factory can affect milk production.

Flat and Inverted Nipples

Your baby is hardwired to seek the firm nipple on the "top of the hill" by rooting and feeling the landscape of the breast with his cheek. A "flat" nipple that doesn't protrude much congenitally or because of postpartum edema is confusing and harder to sense. You can help him sense it more easily by placing your fingers on one side of the breast and your thumb on the other about two inches back from the nipple and compressing lightly to form a "sandwich" that lines up with baby's mouth. Pressing your index finger up into the breast and outward can push some inverted nipples out farther; this technique is informally referred to as the "nipple nudge." This may need to be maintained while baby nurses.

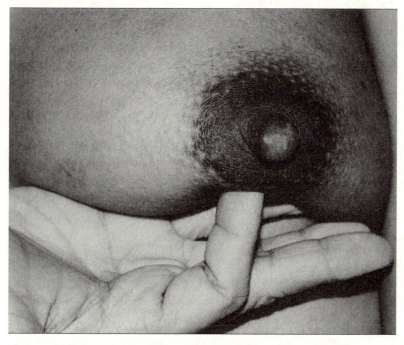

The "nipple nudge" can help push the nipple out and make latching easier.

Around 3 percent of women have congenitally inverted nipples that pull back into the breast. This is caused by either exceptionally short milk ducts or fibrous adhesions that constrict the nipple, drawing it inward. Women with inverted nipples tend to have more problems with milk production, usually because baby has difficulty latching and drawing out milk. In some cases, there may be fewer ducts, or the ducts are obstructed. Occasionally, breasts with inverted nipples may have other structural problems as well.[1]

Some nipples appear inverted, but when the areola directly behind them is gently compressed, they protrude fairly easily. After a few weeks of breastfeeding, they typically remain everted until weaning. True inverted nipples pull inward when the areola behind them is compressed. Of these, some can be manually pulled out, at least momentarily. Others are firmly tethered in the breast and can't be pulled out at all. Both types of true inversions are tricky for babies to learn to attach to, but tethered nipples cause the most problems. They may not drain well or at all, even for a good breast pump. In such cases, little can be done, and the breast will eventually dry up.

Inverted nipples can be surgically released, but only when you are neither pregnant nor lactating. The ability to breastfeed afterward depends on the underlying cause of the inversion, any nerve damage from the surgery, and the healing process. An inversion caused by fibrous adhesions can be released without affecting milk production capability. However, surgery for an inversion caused by short ducts severs the ducts, making it difficult for milk to exit unless they reconnect over time.[2] A nonsurgical option for treating inverted nipples is the Avent Niplette™, which creates sustained suction in a small cup worn inside the bra for several hours at a time. This has been reported to correct both types of inverted nipples but requires at least one to three months, ideally before the last trimester of pregnancy.[3]

Once baby is here, your two goals are to help him latch and to keep the milk moving. First try *reverse pressure softening* if there is any edema (see Chapter 11). Then, see if you can gently pull your nipple out by pushing your fingers deep into your breast and finding the sides or "back" of the nipple shank. You can also use the Maternal Concepts Evert-It™ Nipple Enhancer to do this, or you can use a periodontal syringe with the tip end cut off and the plunger inserted so that the smooth side is against you. Pumping for a minute or two may also draw out the nipple, but this may cause the areola to swell, creating a bulb of tissue that may be too large for baby to latch to. Whichever you try, once you let go, the nipple will usually retract quickly, so you'll have to work fast to get baby latched.

When all else fails, a properly sized silicone nipple shield can create an artificial nipple to help baby latch, so long as your actual nipple can be pulled out a little and isn't tethered. Invert the dome of the nipple shield halfway, then press the flat part of the shield on the areola. The dome should pop back into shape, drawing the nipple partially into it to increase baby's effectiveness. Before baby latches, compress your breast behind the shield to express some milk into the dome to encourage him to suck. (You can also inject milk through a hole with a periodontal syringe.) Make sure he latches as deeply as possible! Finally, pump after feedings to thoroughly drain the breasts because it can be difficult for baby to remove milk effectively with a nipple shield in this situation. A shield is usually temporary until baby learns to trust the breast and latch easily.

Unusually Shaped Nipples

Nipples are generally round and cylindrical but can also come in unusual shapes such as bumpy, elongated, or separated into two distinct parts. Most nipples still work normally, but if they are partially or completely nonfunctional, lack of milk removal usually leads to an unavoidable shutdown in production.

Large Nipples

If you naturally have large nipples or started with normal-sized nipples that enlarged after years of nursing, baby can have trouble latching. When the mismatch is too great, baby can't get his mouth around the nipple and deep enough onto the areola to adequately draw milk. Deanne Francis, B.S.N., IBCLC, wittily refers to this condition as "oro-boobular disproportion." The solution is to feed baby by an alternative method and pump—you'll need extra large flanges—until his mouth grows bigger. Latch him periodically until he can do it comfortably and remove milk well. If he has trouble returning to the breast, see "Breast Refusal" in Chapter 4 or contact a lactation consultant.

Nipple Piercings

Although some babies don't seem to like a breast that has piercing scars, nipple piercings aren't usually a problem for milk production; if anything, they may add additional outlets in the nipples. (Removal of any nipple rings or bars during feedings is recommended, of course.) However, unusual or extensive scarring due to infections or poor piercing technique could obstruct milk flow. If this happens, there isn't anything you can do to fix it; the lobes that can't drain will eventually dry up. Pumping and galactogogues can help you get the most from the usable areas. Areolar piercings can also cause damage to the nerves that affect milk ejection (see Chapters 10 and 11 for methods to stimulate milk ejection).

Breast Structure

Two basic breast structure issues can affect milk production. *Tissue density* is the relative elasticity and compressibility of the breast, areola, and nipple, ranging from very firm to jello-soft. *Glandular development* refers to the overall amount of milk-making tissue.

Soft Breast Tissue

Soft, flaccid breast tissue can be difficult for some babies to grasp. In some instances, the skin is so loosely attached to the underlying gland that baby has mostly skin in his mouth and can't extract milk efficiently. Firmly shaping the breast and pulling back toward your chest wall to tighten the skin against the gland can help baby get his mouth around the milking area. Or try the "nipple nudge" described earlier in this chapter to make the nipple and areola stick out farther. Holding baby against your side with his feet pointing behind you may align him to latch more easily. Breast compressions are usually necessary to remove all of the available milk to keep up your supply.

Insufficient Glandular Tissue

Women with small breasts often worry that they don't have enough milk-making tissue, but smaller breasts don't necessarily mean there's less tissue any more than having large breasts means there's more. It isn't the outer size of the breasts that matters, but rather the amount of glandular tissue inside them. This starts with a healthy basic tree in place before pregnancy and then having that tree respond to the pregnancy with new growth. True insufficient glandular tissue, or *mammary hypoplasia*, usually refers to the state of the breasts before pregnancy and typically involves a lack of fullness in part or all of the breast. Small breasts may look peripubertal, as if they never completed puberty, and are often less than an A cup with little palpable tissue. Larger hypoplastic breasts may look "deflated" or have an unusually long tubular or bowed shape, with the nipples pointing down or away from the body. One side may be much larger than the other, known as asymmetric. There may also be stretch marks that aren't related to pregnancy or adolescent growth.

Decreased development usually results in more flat space between the breasts; greater than 1.5 inches (4 centimeters) is considered higher risk for milk supply problems. The areolas may also be disproportionately large and "bulbous," almost as if they're a separate structure attached to the breast. Most telling, affected women usually experience few, if any, breast changes during pregnancy and have difficulty identifying when the breasts start making milk after birth.[4] However, more mammary growth may occur after birth if there is frequent milk removal and stimulation. The permanence of hypoplasia is discussed in more detail in the next chapter.

A fair question to ask is why some breasts would be hypoplastic at all; it certainly isn't common in nature when survival depends on our ability to nourish our young. Is it congenital? Is it hormonal?

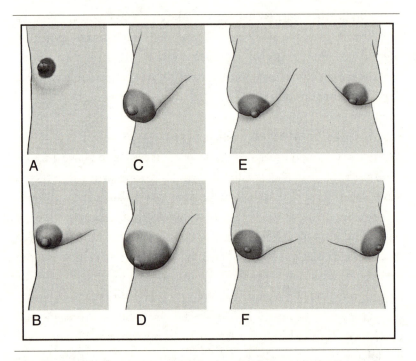

Hypoplasia variations: A—incomplete development before puberty; B—poorly developed upper portion, scant lower tissue; C—tubular with bulbous areola; D—long, bowed to outside, with extra-large areola; E—classic wide-spaced and uneven; F—wide-spaced with scant tissue.

Is there another cause? We simply don't know yet. Some mothers say that their breast shape "runs in the family," which suggests a hormonal-genetic component, while others have no close relatives with hypoplasia. As discussed in Chapter 9, women with polycystic ovary syndrome (PCOS) have hormonal problems that sometimes affect breast development. Breast hypoplasia seems to have been rarer in the past but may now be increasing. Why might this be?

Environmental research may shed light on at least part of this mystery. Common contaminants in our environment can bind in place of regular hormones to hormone receptors, potentially altering normal hormonal function.[5] Exposure to organochlorines, such as TCDD and DDE, or to substances like BPA and PCBs has been found to stunt mammary gland development in rats, and there are reports of poor glandular development or early weaning, presumably due to poor milk production, in women living in heavily exposed areas. In some cases, the breasts looked normal, but the glandular tissue inside was spotty or scant.[6] The less glandular tissue there is, the less milk can be produced. With hard work, many women are able to improve their supplies significantly, while others seem to hit a ceiling quickly.[7] One of the biggest hurdles is getting enough stimulation, since not all babies will continue to suck vigorously when milk flow is low. At-breast supplementation is an ideal strategy to encourage vigorous suckling while simultaneously feeding baby. Breast compression also helps baby drain the breast more thoroughly. Additional pumping after a feeding coupled with more breast compression helps complete breast drainage and provides the extra stimulation that is often needed to continue stimulating hormones and receptors.

Galactogogues can make a difference but are often disappointing, perhaps because expectations tend to be high! The best herbal choices are those that have a dual reputation of also stimulating mammary growth, such as goat's rue (Chapter 12). Prescription galactogogues superstimulate the existing tissue. Good results for either depend in part on how much functional breast tissue there is to work on.

Surgeries

With few exceptions, most mothers who have had breast surgery (either for cosmetic or medical reasons) are able to produce some amount of milk, so the question is not *if* you will produce milk, but rather *how much* milk you will be able to make. This is determined by the amount of damage to the ducts and nerves, the functionality of the milk glands prior to surgery, the healing process, the amount of time since the surgery, and any other lactation experiences between the surgery and current baby. Scarring or the complication of an infection may have an effect on lactation, depending on the extent.

Ducts are able to regenerate over time in response to the stimulation of pregnancy and lactation. If you had a partial milk supply with your first baby, you may find that you get progressively more milk with each subsequent baby, sometimes even a full supply. The subtle stimulation from each menstrual cycle also plays a role in this regeneration process, so the more time between babies, the better.

The number of genetically determined ductal openings in the nipple makes a difference. The average number is nine but can be as few as four.[8] A woman with nine openings can afford to lose a couple when ducts are severed during surgery, and the milk will still be able to get out, but a woman with only four can't afford to lose any because some areas of her breast may no longer have an outlet. There isn't an easy way to know how many openings you have because they're very small and don't drain at the same time.

When your milk comes in around the third or fourth day after birth, you may be warned about a risk of breast infection from the milk behind severed ducts that "has nowhere to go." This is highly unlikely and is almost never seen in reality. Milk that builds up behind the severed ducts triggers production shutdown and involution of the milk-making cells in the immediate area. Meanwhile, the unaffected areas of the breast will continue to function and work even harder so long as milk is removed from them.

Like ducts, nerve fibers can also regenerate. The most critical nerve to lactation is the *fourth intercostal nerve*, which is generally located around the four o'clock position facing the left breast and the eight o'clock position facing the right. It is the primary carrier of messages to the brain for the release of prolactin and oxytocin, and when injured, milk ejection doesn't happen as easily.[9] Unlike ducts, nerve regeneration is *not* influenced by lactation, past or current, but grows at a consistent rate of 0.04 inches (1 millimeter) per month after an initial period of repair. Normal response to touch and temperature indicates that the nerve network is improving, although the healing process can vary, and it's possible that your nipples may never regain all of their previous sensitivity and functionality. The longer it's been since the surgery, the greater the chances that the critical nerves have regenerated to their ultimate potential. Chapter 10 discusses ways to stimulate or enhance milk ejections.

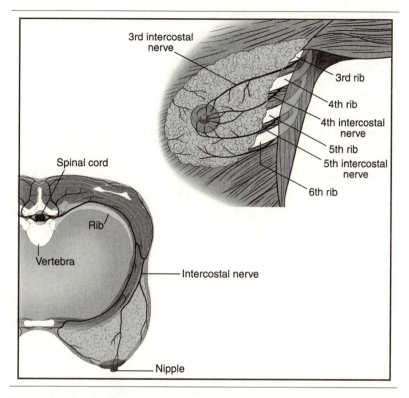

Nerves that directly affect the breast and lactation

Maximizing milk removal, as explained in Chapter 5, is the best initial strategy for ensuring that you make the most milk possible after breast surgery. In most cases, pumping, galactogogues, and strategies to increase milk ejections are also necessary. Thoroughly massaging your breasts both before and during feedings and using breast compressions may move milk through obstructed areas. Massaging and compressing while pumping can also be effective; try leaning over periodically to let gravity help draw the milk out. If you have implants above the muscle, you can avoid the risk of rupture by placing your hand on top of the breast, with your fingers on one side and your thumb on the other. If baby has difficulty latching deeply because the tissue under your areola isn't as full, try the "nipple nudge" illustrated earlier in this chapter as baby latches.

Diagnostic and Surgical Procedures

Biopsies that remove samples of breast tissue, aspirations to remove infectious or suspicious fluids from the breast, and removal of tissue such as lumps have the potential to interfere with lactation, although the impact is usually mild. Ducts or nerves may be severed, depending on where and what direction the surgeon cut. Incisions that are oriented toward the nipple like the spoke of a wheel reduce the likelihood of damaging nerves and ducts.

One of the most vulnerable periods for significant damage from any surgery is prior to puberty when the immature mammary gland is very small. Invasive cuts during that time can interfere with a greater number of ducts and nerves simply because they are closer together, eventually affecting the internal structure of the breast as it matures.[10]

Breast Lift

Breast lift surgery repositions the breasts to reduce sagging without removing breast tissue, resulting in fuller, rounder, and higher breasts. Breast implant surgery is often performed at the same time to further increase breast fullness. Breast lift surgery alone doesn't usually affect milk production because no glandular tissue is removed and the incisions are not usually deep enough to sever critical nerves.

Breast Implants

Breast implants, or *augmentation*, is a common cosmetic procedure undertaken for many reasons: to enhance appearance, to correct abnormalities, or for reconstruction after other breast surgery. Augmentation surgery can affect your milk-making capability depending on the entry location and the placement of the implants. An incision around the areola, particularly in the lower, outer portion, is likely to reduce nerve response to the nipple and areola. A large implant can also reduce nipple and areolar sensitivity.[11] An implant positioned directly under the glandular tissue is more likely to put pressure on the tissue and obstruct milk flow, resulting in reduced milk production over time compared with an implant positioned under the chest muscle away from the tissue.[12] Another important factor to consider is the reason for your surgery. If your breasts were unusual in shape, perhaps lacking the normal amount of glandular tissue, the cause of a low milk supply later on could have more to do with a smaller amount of milk-making tissue than the surgery you had to even them out.

Breast Reduction

Breast reduction surgery reduces milk production capability in most cases because it removes mammary tissue and damages nerves.[13] The techniques that harm production the least are those in which the areolae and nipples are not completely severed, even though they may have been moved, such as in the liposuction and "pedicle" surgeries. With most reduction surgeries, though, there is likely to be some damage to the ducts and nerves as a result of deep cuts in the breast tissue. The amount of milk made after reduction surgery varies tremendously, ranging from very little to full production. For more detailed information about breastfeeding after breast reduction surgery, including descriptions of breast reduction techniques, refer to *Defining Your Own Success: Breastfeeding After Breast Reduction Surgery* by Diana West and visit www .bfar.org (Breastfeeding After Breast and Nipple Surgeries), which also features an online support forum.

Infections

Lactation is a robust process, but when your health is compromised, milk production can suffer as well. Serious infections or conditions, especially life-threatening ones, may cause your body to cut back on production in order to divert more energy into healing. As long as stimulation and milk removal continues, your supply usually comes back as your condition improves. The milk is almost always safe for baby during treatment. On rare occasions, breast tissue damage from abscess, extreme prolonged engorgement, or severe mastitis may account for some otherwise inexplicable cases of low milk production.

Injuries

Various injuries have the potential to interfere with milk production by damaging glandular tissue or critical nerve connections. The types of injuries that are described next are the most likely to cause problems with milk production.

Spinal Cord Injuries

The nerves that supply the breast enter the spinal cord in the middle of the back at the T3, T4, T5, and T6 vertebrae, in the thoracic region.[14] Spinal injuries below this should not affect milk production directly, but injuries above T6 carry the potential to cause problems. A complete injury results in the loss of all motor and sensory function at the level of the injury and below, while an incomplete injury may allow for some sensory or motor function at the level of the injury or below.[15] Spinal cord injuries are a concern for breastfeeding because they interfere with the normal messages sent by the suckling baby to the brain that stimulate the release of prolactin and oxytocin. It has generally been accepted that injuries above T6 usually result in a decrease in milk production between six weeks and three months. But a recent report may shed light on why the decreases occur and what compensations are possible. Three women had neck injuries resulting in paralysis of both lower and upper body. Two were first-time mothers, while the third had successfully breastfed a baby before her injury. In each case their milk came in normally, but milk ejection wasn't consistent. To compensate, some learned to bypass the physical and rely on the secondary emotional pathway of mental imaging and relaxation to elicit milk ejection, often multiple times during the feeding. Oxytocin nasal spray was also used for the same purpose. Both of these strategies helped the babies to get more milk and the mothers to sustain higher milk production for a longer time.[16]

Blunt Force Trauma

Blunt force trauma occurs when the body is suddenly impacted by an object with great force. Breast tissue can be damaged, such as during a bad car accident when a seat belt across the chest crushes the breast and causes bruising. Damage from blunt force trauma may be intensified in young girls and teens whose breasts haven't started or completed development. Imagine dropping a rock on a flower, then dropping the same rock on a flower bud. The fully bloomed flower may be bruised, but not all of it will be harmed. The bud, however, is smaller and more completely crushed, and it may never bloom normally. The potential damage to breast tissue before and after puberty is similar, but each case is individual. If the side you were hurt on has lower milk production, your injury is a likely cause of the problem. This may be a permanent condition, but most mothers should be able to make enough milk with the undamaged breast to compensate. You may find that the higher-producing breast becomes larger because it is doing most of the work. It's a temporary inconvenience that will gradually diminish throughout lactation and weaning.

Burn Trauma

Damage to the breast tissue from burns on your chest varies depending on when it happened, how deep the burn went, and the extent of scarring. If the burn wounds were superficial, scarring is probably the biggest problem, with possible blockage of the nipple pores and poor elasticity of the skin that can make latching more difficult. Deeper wounds may destroy milk-making tissue. Burn injuries to a young girl's chest can damage the undeveloped gland and prevent normal growth later on. A lactation consultant can help you strategize and work around the damage as much as possible.

Muscular-Skeletal Problems

A variety of situations ranging from accidents to repetitive motions can result in subtle muscular-skeletal problems that can impinge nerves and obstruct lymphatic and blood flow, resulting in areas of numbness, tingling, or other unusual symptoms. This may reduce the sensations that trigger hormones, or a kink elsewhere in the nerve pathway might prevent messages from getting to the brain. If you've had such symptoms and your milk supply problem doesn't seem to have another cause, it may be worth exploring the possibility of a mechanical interference with a chiropractor, doctor of Chinese medicine, or other holistic practitioner (see Chapter 11).

CHAPTER 9

Is It Your Hormones?

If you believe that both you and your baby have all the right equipment and yet you aren't making enough milk, what could be going on? It is especially frustrating if well-meaning friends or relatives tell you that you just need to try a little harder, or that maybe you're just too high-strung. Read on! You may find some clues here that will help you solve your personal mystery.

The piece of the equation least addressed by research is the active physiological process of making milk—having the right ingredients and instructions. This refers not to your diet but rather to your *hormones* and their complex interactions that bring everything together and direct milk production.

The Milk Supply Equation

Sufficient glandular tissue

+ Intact nerve pathways *and* ducts

+ **Adequate hormones *and* hormone receptors**

+ Adequately frequent, effective milk removal and stimulation

= GOOD MILK PRODUCTION

Hormonal Issues: The Big Spider Web

Probably the most confusing and confounding aspect of trying to understand problems related to hormonal issues is the many complex interrelationships between conditions. Sometimes the question becomes, "Which came first; the chicken or the egg?" Is the hormone problem the cause of low milk production, or is it a symptom of another issue?

Hormones are complex and difficult to study because they interrelate like a giant spider web. They can affect their own receptors, other hormones, and other hormone receptors. Timing can determine whether lactation is affected or not. For instance, problems with key hormones during the critical window of puberty could affect the developing breast structures, resulting in hypoplasia (see Chapter 8).

Certain conditions that affect various mammary and lactation hormones will be discussed individually in this chapter, but it also helps to look at the big picture as you try to understand what may be askew in your body when milk production doesn't seem to be working right. For instance, if your body doesn't make enough progesterone, it's possible that this could affect the development of your milk factory and your eventual milk supply. A problem with any of the three major milk hormones, prolactin, insulin, and cortisol, could certainly throw a monkey wrench into your milk production machinery. If there is a problem with oxytocin, it could cause a decrease in your ability to release milk, which would automatically lead to decreased milk production.

Actual hormonal deficits are possible, though not common, and in rare instances can be an inherited condition. In one documented case, a mother with no detectable milk also had almost no measurable prolactin, a problem that apparently ran in her family.[1] Prolactin replacement, now being researched, will be helpful when it becomes available.

The receptor side of hormone function has been the neglected element in the Milk Supply Equation, yet having a receptor problem is the same as not having enough hormone because the hormone can't get where it needs to go. At least one study has looked at whether prolactin resistance can happen and interfere with normal milk production.[2] Insulin resistance is certainly known, and cortisol resistance also may not be as rare as previously thought.

Edema

Water retention in the body, called *edema*, is common toward the end of pregnancy. Nurses and lactation consultants report that a growing number of women are now also experiencing water retention and swelling that seems to develop or worsen during and after hospital deliveries. Their breasts may feel hard and swollen to the point that the nipple and areola flatten out as if engorged with milk. So far there is no good research, but some believe that it may be due to intravenous (IV) fluids building up in the body, while others think that Pitocin (artificial oxytocin), which is chemically similar to antidiuretic hormone (ADH), may bind to or increase the number of ADH receptors and temporarily cause more water retention. Whatever the reason, there seems to be a connection between this edema and delayed milk production; often the milk doesn't come in fully until the swelling subsides.

Diuretic drugs are rarely prescribed because edema is usually a self-correcting condition. If you are anxious to speed the process of eliminating the excess water to help your milk come in, there are foods with diuretic properties, such as dandelion greens, dandelion tea, watermelon, cucumbers, asparagus, cabbage, and celery, that you can try, though you'll need to eat a lot of them!

Obesity

Obesity, defined as a prepregnancy body mass index (BMI) greater than twenty-six, is a risk factor for both delayed lactation and low milk production. In animal experiments, overfeeding and excessive weight has been related to poor mammary growth both before and during pregnancy. Research hasn't examined this possibility in humans, but a study of obese mothers who weren't making enough milk found that they often had lower prolactin surges in response to nursing or pumping even though they started with levels similar to nonobese mothers. It's quite possible that mammary gland development during puberty or pregnancy also may be affected in a manner similar to the animal studies, and excessive weight gain during pregnancy could also alter breast growth during that time.[3]

Exploring the underlying cause of obesity may provide additional clues for milk supply problems. Many people assume that obesity is simply the result of overeating, but there are metabolic disorders that affect milk production such as hypothyroidism and polycystic ovary syndrome (PCOS) that also cause weight gain. Obese women also frequently suffer from insulin resistance and diabetes, which are often reversible with weight loss.

Diabetes

The breast is a major consumer of insulin, a key hormone that plays a role in mammary development and milk production. Insulin receptors in the breast are normally somewhat resistant but become more sensitive to insulin during pregnancy in preparation for making milk. Diabetes is a disease or condition in which the body either does not produce enough insulin or does not use it properly. There are two major forms of diabetes.

Type 1 Diabetes

Insulin-dependent diabetes mellitus (IDDM), also known as type 1 diabetes, occurs when the pancreas is unable to manufacture enough insulin to meet the body's needs. As a result, additional insulin is required to make up the deficit. During pregnancy, prolactin and human placental lactogen can be lower in type 1 diabetic mothers, possibly affecting mammary gland development and lactation. As milk production begins after birth, the body's metabolic needs change dramatically, altering insulin requirements. This can slow the milk coming in up to twenty-four hours, depending on how quickly adjustments to insulin replacement are made.[4] Any significant fluctuations in insulin can cause a decrease in milk production at any time during lactation. Tight control of blood sugar and insulin levels can help women with this type of diabetes maintain consistent milk production for baby. Insulin therapy is safe for lactation because the molecule is too large to pass into the milk. Type 1 diabetes may also affect thyroid function, another issue described later.

Type 2 Diabetes

Also called *non-insulin-dependent diabetes mellitus* (NIDDM), type 2 diabetes does not require insulin therapy. Instead, your body makes enough insulin but is not able to use it well because of a problem with receptor binding. The resulting *insulin resistance* creates a "rusty lock" effect that makes getting enough insulin and glucose into the cells more difficult. The body's response is to compensate by increasing insulin production further, resulting in *hyperinsulinemia*. When the effort of overproducing insulin wears the pancreas out, type 1 diabetes results. Insulin receptors naturally become slightly more resistant than usual as a normal process of pregnancy, but when they become too resistant, a temporary form of type 2 diabetes called *gestational diabetes* can occur. Many mothers with type 2 or gestational diabetes make plenty of milk, but some don't. Women with milk supply problems *and* confirmed insulin resistance often have breast hypoplasia as well.[5] More research is needed on the relationship between insulin resistance and breast development.

Hypertension

Hypertension is diagnosed when blood pressure is higher than normal. Mothers who have hypertension before pregnancy are said to have *chronic hypertension*. High blood pressure that starts after twenty weeks gestation is called *gestational hypertension*. *Pregnancy-*

induced hypertension (PIH), also known as *toxemia* or *preeclampsia*, is a form of gestational hypertension accompanied by protein in the urine and sudden swelling of the hands, feet, or face. *HELLP syndrome* (named for its main symptoms: *hemolytic anemia, elevated liver enzymes*, and *low platelet count*) is a severe variation of PIH. Whatever the origin, hypertension is considered a risk factor for poor milk production.[6] The exact mechanism is not well understood, especially because not all women with high blood pressure have difficulty making milk. But it is known that hypertension can affect the placenta, which in turn could affect breast development (see the section "Placental Problems" later in this chapter).[7] Questions also have been raised about the drugs used to treat hypertension, especially in pregnancy, but so far we don't have any definite answers.

Anemia

Anemia, a low red blood cell count, can be an inherited condition or caused by disease, infection, drug exposure, inadequate nutrition, or excessive blood loss. Most cases are related to iron deficiency and may not have obvious signs. Fatigue is the most common symptom, but as anemia becomes progressively worse, weakness, pale skin (especially the inner lining of the eyelids), rapid heartbeat, shortness of breath, chest pain, dizziness, irritability, numbness or coldness in hands and feet, or headache may occur. Mild anemia is common during pregnancy and rarely a problem, but if there is a large loss of blood during delivery, anemia can develop or worsen. Sleep-deprived new mothers may not always realize that anemia may be contributing to their fatigue.[8]

There is some evidence that anemia can affect lactation, though research has been limited. If you have low iron, researchers believe that it's best to treat it whether or not you have obvious symptoms in order to optimize milk production. Share this with your doctor and ask him what he recommends. In the meantime, eat high-iron foods together with food or drinks high in vitamin C to help your body to absorb more iron and rebuild your stores. Galactogogue herbs that contain iron may be useful (see Chapter 12).

Postpartum Hemorrhage and Sheehan's Syndrome

Severe bleeding after delivery can pose two risks to milk production. Most obvious is the large loss of red blood cells and possible anemia. The loss of up to a pint (500 cubic centimeters) of blood with vaginal births and up to 2 pints (1,000 cubic centimeters) with cesarean surgery is considered within normal limits. Higher amounts of blood loss have been associated with poor milk production.

The second risk from postpartum hemorrhage involves the pituitary gland, which enlarges during pregnancy. If there is a sudden loss of a large amount of blood, *hypovolemia* (decrease in blood plasma volume) may ensue and the pituitary gland may collapse. Mild to moderate damage is referred to as a *pituitary insult* and causes reduced functioning, depending on the severity. Severe damage is known as a *pituitary infarction* or *Sheehan's syndrome*. Resulting problems may be immediately obvious or may occur over time, and hypothyroidism eventually occurs in half of all cases of pituitary damage. Prolactin and milk production can be moderately to completely suppressed.[9] Galactogogue drugs that stimulate prolactin can be only as effective as the pituitary's ability to respond. Prolactin replacement therapy, once developed, has the potential to restore milk production.

Mona Gabbay, M.D., IBCLC, a physician with a breastfeeding medicine practice in New York, finds that baseline prolactin levels are often below 30 nanograms per milliliter in mothers who have experienced postpartum hemorrhage and low milk supply. She reports improved milk production with domperidone treatment (see Chapter 12).

Measuring Prolactin

Prolactin is tricky to measure and interpret because it varies depending on your stage of lactation. It's highest around birth and then declines over the next few months to a lower plateau. *Baseline measurements* are those taken when there hasn't been nipple stimulation for at least ninety minutes. Prolactin is lower in the daytime and rises at night during sleep. A *prolactin surge* is the rise *above* the baseline in response to stimulation. Ideally, blood is drawn before a feeding for a baseline measurement and then again forty-five minutes after starting to nurse or pump to measure the surge. In the early months, it will at least double, sometimes reaching ten to twenty times the baseline. Some experts believe that the prolactin response to suckling is more significant than the actual baseline number. If cost prohibits two separate tests, a baseline taken right before feeding is the better choice.

Some women have been told that their prolactin level was normal when in fact it was quite low for lactation. Standard lab reports list only the normal range for nonpregnant, nonlactating females, and physicians may not always remember this. If testing is done while you are taking a prolactin-increasing drug, the results may be much higher than expected, and there will be little or no rise with suckling or pumping.

Appropriate Prolactin Levels

Stage	Baseline (ng/mL)	Level with Suckling (ng/mL)
Female menstrual life	2–20	—
Third trimester of pregnancy	150–250	—
Term pregnancy	200–500	—
First 10 days postpartum	200	400
10 days–3 months	60–110	70–220
3 months–6 months	50	100
6 months–1 year	30–40	45–80

Sources: Cox D, Owens R, Hartmann P. Blood and milk prolactin and the rate of milk synthesis in women. *Exp Physol.* 1996;81(6):1007–20. Lawrence R, Lawrence R. *Breastfeeding: A Guide for the Medical Profession.* 6th ed. Philadelphia, PA: Elsevier Mosby; 2005:75.

Placental Problems

Joan had successfully breastfed two other children, but her third baby, born prematurely due to a separating placenta, was not thriving. She reported that her breasts didn't grow or change much this pregnancy, nor did milk come in well despite excellent management.

Anything that compromises placental function can also affect breast development during pregnancy.[10] A diagnosis of "placental insufficiency" is a red flag, as is any significant separation of the placenta, referred to as *placental abruption*, occurring earlier on, especially if that led to more complications. (A compromised placenta can be the reason a baby is born small for his gestational age.) Poor glandular development caused by a poorly functioning placenta is difficult to remedy, but not impossible; you can still build breast tissue with frequent stimulation by nursing or pumping just as adoptive mothers do. Galactogogues that stimulate breast growth are the best choice in this situation.

Progesterone also may be lower during a pregnancy with placental problems. In rats, this has caused premature labor and sometimes even the start of milk production *before* birth. Involution then began because milk was not being removed; the milk factory literally began to tear down before it even opened for business! There have been a few cases reported of women who had preterm labor followed by engorgement and milk leakage. Once baby was born, their milk did not come in at all. Though not tested, supplemental progesterone therapy at the first sign of placental problems might be able to rescue some of these situations by allowing continued breast development and stopping the premature initiation of full milk production.

A different type of placental problem is retained placenta. Once baby is born and the placenta is delivered, progesterone levels drop rapidly and the milk comes in. On rare occasions, a piece of tissue may break off from the placenta and remain attached to the uterine wall. This will often cause heavy bleeding or even hemorrhaging, so it is usually discovered and treated quickly. But if symptoms are more subtle and the piece stays inside, continued progesterone can interfere with the start-up of milk production. Sometimes lack of milk may be the first clue that a piece of placenta remains. This is more likely to happen in deliveries where the placenta was slow to expel or tension was applied to help the placenta come out. It can even happen with a cesarean delivery.

Marie had previously breastfed four other children, but her new baby was not getting enough milk to grow well. A plan was developed to continue nursing, pumping, and supplementing. Two weeks later, the baby was suddenly gulping milk contentedly at the breast. When asked if there were any significant changes that week, Marie responded, "Well, I did have this really weird thing happen a couple of days ago. I had a lot of cramping and then I passed these big clots. . . ." The improvement in milk production occurred soon after this event. Marie remembered that her obstetrician had kept traction on the umbilical cord until the placenta came out. Case solved.

When a mother's postpartum bleeding is in the normal range but milk production is sluggish to start, Pamela Berens, M.D., suggests ruling out retained placental tissue with a blood test for beta human chorionic gonadotropin (β-hCG), a placental hormone that normally decreases rapidly after birth. A transvaginal ultrasound is another possible screening test; a negative result is usually correct, but a positive result could wrongly interpret post-birth debris as placental tissue. As in Marie's case, retained tissue can clear out on its own, but when identified earlier, it's usually removed surgically to avoid the risk of hemorrhage. Increased milk production usually occurs within forty-eight hours.

In rare cases, a more severe version of placental retention can occur. Rather than merely attaching to the uterine wall, the placenta may grow into the wall and sometimes through the wall and even to other organs. This often causes hemorrhaging because the pieces cannot easily let go and come out after birth. Manual removal of the placenta may be attempted, and medications such as Methergine or methotrexate may be used to help complete the job and control bleeding. These drugs carry some risk of suppressing or reducing milk production, though short-term use is considered less risky.

Your physicians, working in tandem with a lactation consultant, are the best resources to help sort through this difficult problem. However, not all are aware of the connection between the placenta and the start of milk production or may not be open to the possibility because they feel that it implies error on their part. This can make it difficult to receive a serious, thorough evaluation if the symptoms are subtle. You may need a second opinion if your caregiver does not fully explore this possibility with you.

Thyroid Dysfunction

Thyroid hormones come from the butterfly-shaped thyroid gland in your neck and are vital to the proper regulation of lactation hormones. Thyroid function involves a complex interaction between the hypothalamus, pituitary, and thyroid glands. Thyroid-releasing hormone (TRH) from the hypothalamus tells the pituitary when to release thyroid-stimulating hormone (TSH), which directs the thyroid gland in the production of thyroxine (T4) and triiodothyronine (T3). Dysfunctions in this process can affect milk production.[11] Problems with your thyroid gland can be hard to detect and diagnose if the symptoms or lab results are not obvious and straightforward. They can also occur together with other conditions such as polycystic ovary syndrome (PCOS), which is discussed later in this chapter, and even cause PCOS-type symptoms.

Thyroid dysfunctions generally fall into two main categories. *Hyper*thyroidism, most often associated with Graves' disease, involves overproduction of thyroid hormones that is usually caused by an overactivity of the thyroid gland. In *hypo*thyroidism, frequently associated with Hashimoto's disease, the problem is inadequate production of thyroid hormones caused by underactivity of the thyroid gland. *Postpartum thyroiditis*, or *postpartum thyroid dysfunction*, often doesn't show up until some time after baby is born. Little research exists on the effects of hypothyroidism and hyperthyroidism on human lactation, but animal research provides some insights.

Hypothyroidism

This is diagnosed when there are high levels of TSH and low levels of T3/T4 (thyroid hormones), typically slowing metabolism and causing weight gain and even depression. Hypothyroidism may exist before pregnancy but occurs for the first time during pregnancy in a small percentage of women. Slightly lower levels of thyroid hormones are normal during pregnancy because some go to the developing baby. This isn't usually a problem, but if you're already hypothyroid, this additional burden can make your condition worse. Untreated hypothyroidism can cause pregnancy-induced hypertension, preeclampsia, placental abruption, anemia, postpartum hemorrhage, and low birth weight. For this reason, hypothyroid mothers are usually monitored carefully, and their medication is often increased during pregnancy. Until recently, it was believed that hypothyroidism affected only milk synthesis, but rat research suggests that poor milk ejection due to impaired oxytocin may be another problem. Poorly controlled hypothyroidism during pregnancy may also reduce the amount of good fats normally manufactured during pregnancy for making milk after baby comes.[12]

Not all thyroid problems show up with the usual tests. Women with low milk production and "low normal" thyroid levels may not be treated because their levels aren't considered low enough. Some women whose TSH and T3 are considered normal, even though they don't feel well, are eventually diagnosed with *subclinical hypothyroidism* by more thorough testing. It can be difficult to find a provider who will pursue borderline cases, so you may need to be persistent. Mothers treated during pregnancy should have their thyroid checked within a couple weeks after birth and again a few weeks later. Hormone needs often decrease after birth, and if medications are not quickly adjusted, this can lead to overmedication and hyperthyroidism, which can also be a problem for milk supply.

Hyperthyroidism

This is diagnosed when TSH is low and T3/T4 are high, and it causes accelerated metabolism and weight loss. Hyperthyroidism occurs less commonly in pregnancy than hypothyroidism. If you were already hyperthyroid, you will usually experience improvement because baby takes some of your hormone, pulling you closer to normal. As a result, you may need less suppressing medication during pregnancy, though symptoms usually rebound shortly after birth. Poorly controlled hyperthyroidism can cause premature delivery, preeclampsia, and fetal growth restriction.

Studies of rats hyperthyroid during pregnancy show multiple problems. First, while they had rapid mammary gland growth, they also were using up mammary fat stores before birth, affecting the amount left to make milk. Second, they had lower prolactin and oxytocin levels during lactation. Because of significant problems with milk ejection, little or no milk came out, depending on the severity of the hyperthyroidism.[13]

There are no published human case reports of hyperthyroidism affecting lactation, but Christine Betzold, NP, IBCLC, M.S.N., from California tells of two mothers with whom she has worked. The first had been hyperthyroid for several years and had a history of good breast growth during pregnancy but premature delivery, severe engorgement, and mastitis with her first two children. Her third baby was also born prematurely, and although she tried to pump, not a drop of colostrum or milk ever came out. She tried galactogogues, but still nothing came out, so she stopped. The second mother had successfully breastfed her first two children, though she had a history of toxemia with each one. During her third pregnancy, she became very hyperthyroid and experienced severe hypertension along with other serious complications that forced a very premature delivery. She didn't start pumping for almost two weeks but also never saw a drop of milk. Both of these mothers had pregnancy and lactation experiences that strongly resemble the rat research. It must be mentioned that a few isolated cases of hyperlactation in hyperthyroid mothers have been informally reported as well. If occurring as postpartum thyroiditis, it's possible that increased metabolism may drive high production because the breast was not affected during pregnancy, but until we have more detailed information, we can't fully explain the paradox.

Postpartum Thyroiditis

Postpartum thyroid dysfunction (PPTD) occurs in up to 7.5 percent of all pregnancies. Type 1 diabetes or smoking (especially more than twenty cigarettes per day) triples this risk. Diagnosis of PPTD often takes time because it can take different patterns. It may start with hyperthyroidism that lasts for a few to several weeks and then transition to hypothyroidism that continues for a few to several months. In some cases, the hyperthyroid stage starts just days after birth, accompanied by severe hypertension. But PPTD can also start with hypothyroidism and change to hyperthyroidism, or it can stay just one or the other. When hyperthyroidism occurs first, it is often not caught until the swing to the hypothyroid phase, which has more obvious symptoms. Even when postpartum hyperthyroidism is detected, many doctors will treat only the hypothyroid phase if it occurs.

Galactogogues may be helpful but probably won't make much difference if the thyroid dysfunction isn't corrected at the same time. For herbal galactogogues, consider those that are reputed to support thyroid function or help with milk ejection (see Chapter 12).

Testing for Thyroid Problems

What's a normal thyroid level? This is currently under debate, with some experts leaning toward tightening the range for TSH from 0.5–5 mIU/L (milli-international units per liter) to 0.5–2.5 mIU/L for preconception and pregnancy.[14] This may be better for lactation as well. Each individual has her own unique hormone profile that doesn't always fit the standards, so explain your concerns to your doctor and ask for an in-depth assessment.[15]

Infertility

A long-standing assumption has been that if a woman can become pregnant, lactation should follow successfully as well. But is this really the case? There has been surprisingly little professional discussion as to whether infertility could be related to low milk production, even though lactation consultants consider it a risk factor.

Causes of infertility vary, of course. When it's related to an underlying hormonal issue on your side, there is potential for interference with breast development before or during pregnancy, or with the milk-making process after delivery. Quite often infertility treatments don't directly correct a problem but "leapfrog" over it to achieve pregnancy. The breasts are ignored, yet they may be missing some of the materials needed to build your milk factory. If you had difficulty getting pregnant and haven't found any other reasons for your low milk production, try to learn as much about the cause of your infertility as possible. Any clues you collect could give you a starting point for what might be wrong and then what you might be able to do about it, as you'll read next.

Polycystic Ovary Syndrome (PCOS)

Polycystic ovary syndrome (PCOS) affects up to 15 percent of all women and is considered the leading cause of female infertility. It seems to be on the rise at the same time that milk supply problems in general appear to be increasing. Many women with PCOS have good milk supplies, and some even complain of overproduction, but PCOS mothers seem to struggle with low milk supply more often than other women do.

PCOS often causes higher levels of androgens (male hormones), estrogen, cholesterol, and insulin (due to insulin resistance); it also causes lower progesterone (due to lack of ovulation) and disrupts other reproductive hormones as well. Hypothyroidism may also be present.[16]

These hormonal problems cause numerous symptoms. High levels of male hormones can result in excess body hair growth, male-pattern balding, and persistent acne. Insulin resistance may cause brown, velvety patches of skin located around the neck, underarms, and groin area, and women with PCOS often develop type 2 diabetes in their thirties and forties. Half of women with PCOS are obese, which may be related to problems with carbohydrate metabolism. Infrequent ovulation is common, which in turn may cause ovarian cysts, irregular menstrual cycles, endometriosis, infertility, and miscarriage. Pregnancy complications such as hypertension, gestational diabetes, preeclampsia, and preterm birth occur more frequently in women with PCOS, who also seem more vulnerable to depression as a result of their hormonal imbalances. Because PCOS is a syndrome rather than a disease, every case is unique and any combination of problems can be found, making diagnosis tricky. For this reason, some health care providers skip the formality of a diagnosis and simply treat the patient's individual problems and symptoms.

A connection between PCOS and milk supply problems was first proposed in a case study of three women with low milk production and common symptoms of PCOS.[17] Researchers have largely overlooked the breast in women with PCOS, but over the years a few have written about underdevelopment of the glandular tissue within the breast, underdevelopment of the outward appearance of the breast, and both. They also mention women who had very large breasts that "simulated [excessive growth]" yet were mostly filled with fat, rather than glandular, tissue.[18] *These findings do not apply to all women with PCOS* but are significant for PCOS mothers with breastfeeding problems.

How might PCOS affect milk production? If the symptoms start very early, around the time of a girl's first period, the breast development that normally happens during puberty may be arrested, especially when the menstrual cycle is never established, resulting in hypoplasia. A lack of normal breast growth during pregnancy is also possible, though whether due to hormonal interference during pregnancy or simply from not starting with enough glandular tissue is uncertain. There is also the possibility that sufficient glandular tissue may be present but hormonal problems are interfering with the normal milk-making process.

To date, two retrospective studies have looked at PCOS and milk production. The first, conducted in the United States, concluded that PCOS didn't cause a higher rate of milk supply problems than that of the general population. However, all the mothers had metformin therapy during the first trimester of pregnancy and some longer, which could positively affect their outcome (discussion coming up). Also, results from PCOS mothers who gave birth prematurely or had multiples, and who may have had more hormonal problems than the average PCOS mother, were excluded.[19]

The second, and most recent, study looked at thirty-six mothers with PCOS and ninety-nine non-PCOS control mothers in Norway, a country with excellent support and high breastfeeding rates.[20] Half of the PCOS mothers were given 1,700 milligrams of metformin daily during pregnancy, and the other half none; the medication was stopped after birth. At one month, 75 percent (27) of the PCOS mothers were exclusively breastfeeding versus 89 percent (88) of the non-PCOS mothers, a 14 percent difference. Five PCOS mothers but only two control mothers did not breastfeed at all. By three months, breastfeeding rates were equal between the two groups. The researchers also discovered a mild negative relationship between third-trimester pregnancy levels of DHEAS, a "pre-androgen," and breastfeeding rates for PCOS mothers, providing a clue to one hormonal problem that might interfere with milk production. They did not look at other hormones besides androgens.

If you have PCOS and are struggling to produce enough milk, first make sure that the problem isn't something else easier and more obvious. If PCOS really seems to be the only explanation, pumping and galactogogues (see Chapter 12 for more information on the galactogogues mentioned here) help in some situations, but quite often aren't enough. Identifying and addressing underlying hormonal problems such as insulin resistance, high androgens, low prolactin levels, or thyroid problems is likely to result in the greatest milk production capability. Metoclopramide is probably not a good idea for depression-prone mothers with PCOS, but domperidone may help get more from your breasts.

One medication being explored for increasing milk production is metformin, which improves PCOS symptoms for many women even when they aren't insulin resistant.[21] There has been informal feedback that it has helped some women significantly, some modestly, and some not at all. Dosages vary, typically starting at 500 milligrams and working up to 1,000 to 2,500 milligrams daily; if you have taken metformin previously, ask your doctor about trying the dosage that was initially needed to improve your symptoms. Metformin during pregnancy reduces the incidence of miscarriage, gestational diabetes, pregnancy-induced hypertension, and premature delivery.[22] It may also reduce hormonal interferences and has been reported by one infertility specialist to improve pregnancy breast growth and lactation for many of his patients.

Goat's rue is one herb that seems especially appropriate for PCOS-related low milk production. It contains galegin and is the herb from which metformin was originally developed. Saw palmetto is reputed to reduce excessive body hair, a symptom of high testosterone. One PCOS mother who tried saw palmetto reported a tripling of her low milk production. Chasteberry has long been used for PCOS and for milk production, and a few PCOS mothers feel it has helped them, but it must be dosed carefully by an herbal practitioner as too much may decrease prolactin.

If you haven't been diagnosed with PCOS but think that perhaps you may have it, a good place to start is a checklist on the website for the Polycystic Ovarian Syndrome Association, www.pcosupport.org/support/quiz.php. Be sure to share your results with your physician, who can help you determine whether or not you have PCOS.

Luteal Phase Defect

Luteal phase defect (LPD) is a condition in which the second half of a woman's monthly menstrual cycle does not proceed normally, and it is another common cause of infertility. As a result of its effect on the menstrual cycle, not enough progesterone is produced. LPD is to blame for many pregnancies that are confirmed early but lost in the days or weeks after the period was due to start.

One reported case of low milk supply was attributed to insufficient mammary gland tissue.[23] When the mother had difficulty conceiving another baby, she was diagnosed with luteal phase defect. After being treated with natural progesterone suppositories from ovulation until twelve weeks into the pregnancy, her milk supply came in normally, and she was able to provide milk fully for her second baby.

When deficiencies exist, extra progesterone throughout pregnancy may allow breast tissue to develop more normally, resulting in better milk production (see Irene's story in Chapter 16). Unfortunately, progesterone will not help after the baby is born because of its role in suppressing milk production during pregnancy.

Gestational Ovarian Theca Lutein Cysts

Your ovaries produce some testosterone, and a small amount is normally present during pregnancy. Rarely, an ovarian cyst called a *gestational ovarian theca lutein cyst* (GOTLC) may develop during pregnancy and secrete up to 10 to 150 times the normal amount. Some women experience a dramatic increase in body or facial hair, balding at the temples, deepening of the voice, or an enlarged clitoris, but if symptoms are mild or absent, the condition may not be noticed and the diagnosis may be missed completely unless your ovaries are inspected during a cesarean surgery or tubal ligation. The cure for GOTLC is birth, after which testosterone levels gradually decline without treatment.

We've known that high levels of testosterone can suppress milk production by interfering with prolactin, but the fact that GOTLC can interfere with milk production was only recently recognized. If you and your caregivers are not aware of the possibility, you may give up too early, assuming that you're "one of those mothers who just can't make enough milk."[24] This is a good reason to have your testosterone checked when there aren't any other explanations. The milk will come in so long as breast stimulation by baby or pump is continued until your testosterone level has dropped low enough. In four reported cases, that was around 300 nanograms per deciliter and took two to four weeks.

Menstruation

Mothers sometimes complain of lower milk production prior to or during their periods, once their cycles have returned. This hasn't been formally studied, but Patricia Gima, IBCLC, reports that a daily dose of 500 to 1,000 milligrams of a calcium/magnesium supplement has helped several of her clients, often within twenty-four hours. Gima recommends taking the supplements from ovulation (midcycle) through about three days into menstruation.

Before jumping to the conclusion that your periods are causing your low milk production, keep in mind that the return of menstruation may actually be a *symptom* and not a cause. A drop in the number of breastfeedings a day or long periods without stimulation (such as baby sleeping through the night) can trigger the return of menstruation. Hormonal birth control can also artificially induce periods in a nursing mother before she might otherwise have started. We don't understand all of the hormonal changes during lactation that cause a woman's body to resume ovulation, but *one of the results of low production can be the return of menstruation*. Did your milk production decrease *before* your periods came back, or after? If it decreased beforehand, then low production triggered the periods, not the other way around. A second question is whether you believe your production drops immediately prior to and during menstruation or if it is low all the time. If it's consistently low, then your period isn't the likely cause.

The Age Factor

The relationship between age and milk production has often been debated but studied very little. There are plenty of mothers in their later thirties or forties (and sometimes beyond) who make lots of milk for their babies. On the other hand, there are also older mothers who have had problems with milk production with no apparent explanation. Most perplexing are the cases of women who previously breastfed other children and then find themselves facing inexplicable low milk production for the first time.

At age forty-two, eight years after the birth of her fifth child, Laura gave birth to Janette. For the first time in her life, Laura struggled with milk production. Her lactation consultant noted that Janette's suck was weak, though it was unclear whether this was due to not getting enough milk or because of a true sucking problem. Pumping and herbal galactogogues were begun, and milk production rose slowly, but still not enough. Laura decided to try domperidone, and finally her supply reached and then surpassed Janette's needs. It became clear over time that Laura's breasts weren't functioning as enthusiastically as they had with her other children and needed a boost.

A key question to ask first is, "What are the surrounding circumstances of the baby's birth?" Is this your first baby after fertility problems or years of health or hormonal problems, or did you simply wait until now to have a baby for other reasons? If the new baby was conceived in the midst of long-term health or reproductive problems, those factors—not age directly—may be the culprit. However, the problem could also be the reverse: health or reproductive problems could be the natural result of an aging process that is now extending to milk production as well.

The high fertility that nature programs into younger women slowly but progressively wanes as we enter our thirties and forties. We all age at different rates, and menopause, the natural end of the fertility road, can happen anywhere from the late thirties to the mid-fifties. Preceding this is *perimenopause*, a time of hormonal fluctuation as the body prepares for this change. The effects of approaching menopause catch up to some of us sooner than others, perhaps causing some problems making enough milk. On the other hand, women who are past menopause have been known to relactate for a grandchild! And mothers who are nursing at the time of a complete hysterectomy, the removal of uterus and ovaries, have continued to nurse uneventfully. These facts cast some doubt on the theory that hormonal changes due to menopause are the key problem.

Another intriguing possibility is the effects of aging itself. Some researchers believe that hormone receptors become resistant to binding with their own hormones as we age. Might this be an issue when older nursing mothers experience low milk supply?

What Do I Do Now?

You may have identified yourself in one or more of the scenarios that were discussed in this chapter. Now what do you do? Read the chapters on increasing milk production so that you know all your options. Then, if needed, discuss your concerns with your health care practitioners and share the relevant parts of this chapter. In some offices, a nurse practitioner may have more time to explore your concerns. Finally, share this information with a skilled lactation consultant so she can help you sort through your options and decide which plan is best for you and your baby.

CHAPTER 10

Can Your Mind Affect Your Supply?

Throughout history, a mother's state of mind has been considered very influential on milk production. This is reflected in the popular wisdom of many cultures, where it is common to hear the warning, "Don't upset a nursing mother or her milk will dry up." Similarly, many "nervous mothers" have been told they won't make enough milk because they're too "high-strung." You may even have heard, "It's all in your head." While making milk is not *all* in your head, your thoughts and feelings *do* play a role in the bigger picture.

Mind over Milk or Milk over Mind?

The brain is wired in such a way that the nerve pathways for milk ejection run through the emotion-processing area of the brain. As a result, the responsiveness of your milk ejection reflex can sometimes be influenced by your emotional state or thought processes. A positive example of this is the way your breasts may start leaking when you hear your or another baby's cry. Your maternal instinct responds to this basic cue and wants to nourish the child in need. On the other side of the coin is the self-conscious new mother nursing in public for the first time. Worried about drawing unwanted attention, she may experience slowed milk ejection, which may cause baby to fuss in protest and draw the attention she feared.

Research on oxytocin, the hormone of milk ejection as well as love and bonding, is still in its infancy. Not only is oxytocin subject to dual sources of physical and emotional stimulation, but it influences other hormones and is in turn influenced by them. Oxytocin influences prolactin, and prolactin may also play a role in the release of oxytocin.[1] We don't know how important this interrelationship is, but it's possible that problems with oxytocin could affect production in subtle ways beyond milk removal.

As we explore how the mind can affect milk production, remember that your body is wired with overlapping "fail-safes" to help you succeed. The very fact that oxytocin release can be triggered through both nipple stimulation and thoughts or feelings shows that nature recognizes the importance of milk ejection. On top of that, the frequent surges of oxytocin from breastfeeding actually have a calming effect, making us less reactive to stress. If lactation was as fragile as many people seem to believe, the human race would never have survived. So as you consider the subtle role of the mind as a possible factor, keep in mind that nature wants you to succeed!

Potential Inhibitors of Milk Ejection

Phyllis was a high school teacher who had carefully prepared for her return to work. On her first day back, however, she called in a panic, reporting that very little milk was coming out when she tried to pump. Further conversation revealed that the curtains had been removed from Phyllis's office, and she felt like a fish in a bowl on display for all the students walking by. No wonder she couldn't pump milk! Once they discussed how to create more privacy, the milk started flowing and everything proceeded normally.

In this situation, Phyllis was worried that she was losing her milk, when in fact she was experiencing a temporary inhibition of her milk ejection reflex. Such short-term episodes rarely have a lasting impact on milk production. However, *chronic* long-term inhibition could reduce production over time because when less milk is removed on a regular basis, less milk is made in the long run. Had Phyllis not changed her uncomfortable environment, her milk supply might have been affected.

Unlike the more tangible physical or management-related causes of low milk production, the impact of psychological inhibition often lessens once it is identified. In most cases, it is possible to work through it by identifying or facing your stressors to understand them better and then making changes when necessary, such as Phyllis creating a more private environment. Even if the issues remain, understanding them will help you feel more in control, which may itself reduce your stress and allow the milk to flow more easily.[2]

Painful Breastfeeding

Breastfeeding shouldn't hurt! Chronic or severe pain while nursing can be a shock and a surprise, something to postpone as long as possible. One mother told her lactation consultant, "I actually put my finger in to check her mouth—I was sure she had some sharp metal razor blades in there." This mother understandably dreaded feedings even though she really wanted to breastfeed. The anticipation of pain can slow milk ejection temporarily, and inhibition can become chronic if breastfeeding is not fixed. When pain is an element of a low supply situation, it's important to get help.

Birth Trauma

Childbirth is good work, but it's often very hard work as well. At times, a difficult birth may become traumatic. Any severe psychological trauma that is related to the baby has the rare but possible potential to spark fear-related inhibition. Cynthia Good Mojab, M.S., IBCLC, a clinical counselor who specializes in the emotional needs and experiences of breastfeeding mothers, explains that a mother may be traumatized if she felt intense helplessness, terror, or horror during birth because she feared for her or her baby's life, or if she experienced or witnessed serious injury during delivery. Birth may bring back memories of abuse or assault in childhood or adulthood. Or labor and delivery may have been challenging and joyous—yet circumstances surrounding birth, such as a family tragedy, may still have left you feeling traumatized.

The reasons may be varied, but the result is the same. A phenomenon that is beginning to be discussed is *post-traumatic stress disorder* (PTSD) due to childbirth, which is estimated to happen following 1.5 percent to 6 percent of all births.[3] PTSD can occur alone, or simultaneously with depression or another psychological disorder. It may also be confused with other disorders such as generalized anxiety disorder. Because experiencing trauma is subjective and women are not routinely screened during pregnancy and labor or after birth, caretakers may not realize that a mother has been traumatized, let alone understand how much time may be required for recovery.

Women who suffer from PTSD related to childbirth may experience nightmares or flashbacks, reliving whatever traumatized them again and again. Two frequent themes are the perception of extreme pain and a sense of loss of control. It is also common to feel emotional detachment from the event or family members and to be anxious and irritable, with outbursts of anger. Places and things that never bothered you before may suddenly trigger fear, putting you constantly on guard. Concentration and memory may be affected, and you may feel as if you are in a daze and life is not real. Emotions may be numb with little or no conscious love felt for your baby or for other family members and friends. This may even extend to a vague discomfort when simply holding or breastfeeding your baby. You may find yourself going through the motions of mothering but feel secretly relieved when others take over care of the baby. You may also experience intense guilt for your detachment. Fearful of reliving the memories, you may avoid the place at which the birth occurred and switch doctors. The normal lack of sleep that comes with parenting a newborn may be compounded by insomnia. Such symptoms may begin immediately or months or even years after the traumatic event.

Recognizing what is happening to you is the first step. Many people who have experienced a traumatic event find it helpful to seek assistance from a mental health professional who is trained in women's trauma issues. Search for someone who is knowledgeable about both trauma recovery and the importance of breastfeeding; ask your lactation consultant or a local La Leche League Leader whom she can recommend. Ideally, this person will be committed to treating you and your baby as an inseparable unit to be supported. *Medications and Mothers' Milk* by Thomas Hale, Ph.D., is an excellent resource for evaluating any medications that may be suggested.

Grief and Loss

Judy contacted a La Leche League Leader because her baby was not doing well at the breast. He would latch easily and suck well but then fuss and didn't seem to get much, even though she was clearly full of milk. Judy was encouraged to pump while continuing to work on breastfeeding and found that she was able to pump plenty of milk. This made the Leader wonder why the baby wasn't able to transfer milk as easily. Following a hunch during a follow-up call, she gently asked her how she felt about being a mother. Judy burst into tears and shared that she was feeling guilty and unworthy of her new baby because of an abortion she had when she was younger. They talked about her pent-up feelings, and a referral was made for more in-depth help. Several days later, Judy called excitedly to say that baby had started feeding at the breast. To her delight, the milk had begun to flow easily, and baby was able to nurse to satisfaction.

The loss of a baby, whether by miscarriage, abortion, stillbirth, disease, SIDS, or accident, is a profound loss in anyone's life. In Judy's case, she had suppressed remorse for a decision in her youth that was brought to the surface by the birth of her new baby, and that burden was subconsciously inhibiting her milk ejection as a consequence. Once she acknowledged her hidden feelings and shared them openly, she was able to shed her burden and move more fully into her role as a nurturing mother.

Loss, especially loss that occurs suddenly and without warning, can be a great shock. We all deal with traumatic experiences differently, and at times nursing mothers have reported "drying up" that was more likely the inhibition of milk ejection. Such a reaction is usually temporary and doesn't have to mean the end of breastfeeding. The best thing is to keep your baby close as you grieve and process your loss. It's not uncommon for well-meaning people to offer to take him in the mistaken belief that this will reduce your stress. What they don't understand is that babies can bring comfort and healing, and milk will soon flow again if nursing is maintained rather than put off.

History of Sexual Abuse

This is one topic that is often glossed over because of our discomfort with the idea, but it has potential to affect breastfeeding. The following story illustrates the complexity of the human mind in coping with conflicting emotions.

Jean contacted a lactation consultant while pregnant with her fourth child. With her first three children, Jean's milk came in, and her breasts felt very full, but the milk did not come out, either for the babies or a pump. So she fed them formula but wanted to try nursing again with her fourth. While asking Jean about her experiences with her other babies, the lactation consultant learned that she had not experienced spontaneous labor with any of them, requiring induction with Pitocin each time. A previous consultant had raised the possibility that Jean had an oxytocin deficit, but because laboratory tests for oxytocin are uncommon, this could not be confirmed. Further questions revealed that Jean had experienced severe sexual abuse as a child that continued into adulthood with an emotionally abusive marriage. Jean consciously worked very hard as a parent to overcome the effects of her horrible childhood, yet it seemed clear that somewhere deep down, her mind and body were reacting to a past that she had not yet resolved. Once baby came, the same scenario repeated itself. Jean later sought counseling, and it was the opinion of her therapist, who had dual expertise in lactation and psychology, that the sexual abuse issues most likely did negatively influence her oxytocin release and milk ejection and possibly affected her birthing as well. Hormone-releasing inhibitions as deep-seated as Jean's are rare but do occur. Help for Jean came after she had completed her family, but she wished she could have worked on her issues beforehand.

Unlike Jean, who was very comfortable with the concept of breastfeeding on a conscious level, some mothers are deeply uncomfortable with the intimacy of breastfeeding and may not realize that it is a disturbing past physical experience that underlies the anxiety they now feel. If you have been sexually abused, your natural concern for your baby's health may be overshadowed by feelings of revulsion when he suckles at your breasts. You may also believe that the baby is rejecting you if he has difficulty latching or fusses when your milk flow is slow.

The experience of abuse may be only vaguely remembered. It may not even have been an actual sexual encounter so much as a physically threatening intimacy. In rare cases, a long-suppressed memory may evoke old feelings of threat or panic even though you cannot recall anything specific. Counseling may eventually reveal the underlying roots. A healthy breastfeeding relationship can help a mother become comfortable with intimacy and human touch again, providing the opportunity to work through feelings and experience a greater degree of healing.

Abusive Partner

A woman who is being battered by her partner is also a trauma victim. During crisis, adrenaline begins to flow as her body goes into self-protective "fight-or-flight" mode. From nature's standpoint, survival of the mother ranks higher than survival of the baby, and the body will inhibit other processes, including the delivery of milk to the baby, under such circumstances. When the danger has passed, milk will flow more easily again, but frequent battering could lead to chronic, extreme stress that in turn could affect milk production over time. If you are experiencing physical abuse, you *must* get help for your and your baby's safety.

Harnessing Your Mind to Make More Milk

Are you dismayed to discover that your mind can affect your milk ejection? Don't be, because this can be turned around to your advantage! By harnessing your thoughts, it's possible to use your mind to stimulate more milk ejections, which allows baby to remove more milk and stimulate higher production. For some mothers, this may be very powerful, resulting in a considerable increase in flow. For others, particularly those for whom milk production is low due to secondary reasons, psychological techniques may not have a great effect. Either way, it may be worthwhile to see if any of the following ideas strike a chord. Meanwhile, the deep relaxation will be beneficial.

The methods described are useful for both mothers who have experienced problems with milk ejection as a result of severe psychological stress as well as mothers who would like to explore psychological tools as an additional way to stimulate milk production. But keep in mind that these are meant to be used *along with frequent, adequate milk removal.* If milk is not being drained fully from the breast, no technique to improve milk production can be effective.

Create a Relaxing Environment

Your environment is important to your feeling of safety and peace. When you're breastfeeding or pumping, try to minimize negative elements in your immediate surroundings. This may mean moving to a quiet room away from the rest of the family, especially anyone who is not entirely supportive of breastfeeding. Put on some music if you find it relaxing. Before you begin, take a few slow, deep breaths to clear your mind and body of any remaining tension. The influence of your environment on milk release is a factor that can change over time. Confidence is built with experience, and soon your mind will work effortlessly and efficiently in the busyness of day-to-day life.

Nurture Yourself

Do you find it difficult to relax? "Self-care" measures help you to relax more fully so that milk ejections come as easily as possible. Small treats like a nice hot cup of herbal tea, a bubble bath, or a hot shower when someone else is able to take over caring for the baby for a short while can help replenish emotional energy. Or you might find that it is soothing to get out in the fresh air and take a walk. Even stepping outside, looking up, and taking a few deep breaths of fresh air can make a difference. It is amazing how helpful even a few moments of self-care can be.

Distraction

Talking on the phone to supportive friends, reading books and magazines, watching television, and listening to the radio or music while nursing or pumping can be wonderfully effective in facilitating milk ejection by taking your mind off how much milk you are producing or how long the nursing/pumping session has lasted. It can also serve to ease stress and relax your tension.

Condition Your Milk Ejection

Milk ejection can be conditioned to occur in response to a stimulus that you create through a routine. For example, sipping on a special beverage while you nurse may eventually be connected in your mind to breastfeeding, resulting in a milk ejection response whenever you drink it or perhaps even think about it. You can also learn to actively cause milk ejections by noticing what triggers them and then mentally picturing the trigger happening. For instance, if your baby's cry is a trigger for you, then imagine that you hear your baby crying to be fed. Some mothers find that a more abstract image, such as a waterfall, helps to trigger a rush of milk. The more vividly you use your imagination to re-create the physical or emotional sensation of the trigger, the easier it will become to stimulate your milk ejection response.

Visualization has been used to trigger milk ejections even when primary nerves have been damaged. The mothers with spinal cord damage in that fascinating case study discussed in Chapter 8 used mental imagery to induce milk ejection, resulting in significantly increased milk flow: One of the mothers in the study ". . . always breastfed in a quiet location that had no distractions. She began by counting to relax and then by mentally cycling through a series of images and thoughts that most commonly involved thoughts of loving and nurturing her infant. She reported recycling these image patterns several times in the months that she breastfed, because they became less effective if used for several days in a row. Also she reported finding it useful to intersperse the periods of inducing [milk ejection] with a distracting task, such as reading or watching television. Finally, she reported becoming better at inducing [milk ejection] [with her third child] such that she could tolerate some distractions."[4]

Relaxation

The very relaxation techniques that helped you cope through childbirth can now also help your milk to flow! There are two basic methods: physical relaxation and psychological relaxation. With the first, you concentrate on progressively relaxing all the muscles in your body from your toes to your scalp, while breathing deeply. The resulting deep muscular relaxation calms and clears the mind of concern, worry, aggravation, and stress. The second technique starts with the mind, allowing the physical relaxation to follow naturally. Envision anything that gives you a feeling of peace and well-being, such as lying in the sun or sitting beside a mountain lake. Additional physical and psychological relaxation techniques can found on our website at www.lowmilksupply .org/relaxation.

Auditory narratives that provide guided relaxation have been shown to increase milk production.[5] There are several audio CDs that have been developed for this purpose: *Hypnosis for Making More Milk* by Robin Frees, B.A., IBCLC (www.newbornconcepts .com); *Letting Down* by James Wierzbicki and Betsy Feldman (Wil-

low Music); *A Bond Like No Other* by Anji, Inc. (www.anjionline
.com); *Breastfeeding Meditation* by Sheri Menelli (www.menelli.com/
whp/products.htm); and *Pumping Secrets* by Jenniffer Milone (www
.pumpingsecrets.com).

Self-Talk

While learning to relax is an important part of helping milk ejection to happen, there are also other ways to use your mind to get
the same results. One method in particular, known as "self-talk,"
is based on the principle that we all have an ongoing internal dia-
logue. For example, when waking up in the morning, we think,
"I really don't want to get out of bed. I'm tired and I don't want to
change one more diaper." Or, at the end of an enjoyable evening at
the movies, "That was fun! I should get out more often."

Self-talk can be positive or negative and is influenced by
what we hear around us and choose to internalize. Negative self-
statements are usually in the form of phrases that begin like these:
"I just can't do . . ."; "If only I could or didn't . . ."; "I just don't
have the energy. . . ." This type of self-talk represents the doubts
and fears we have about ourselves in general and about our abilities
to deal with discomfort in particular. In fact, negative self-talk can
worsen symptoms like pain, depression, and fatigue.

What we say to ourselves plays a role in determining our success or failure in becoming good self-managers. Learning to make
self-talk work *for* you instead of *against* you can help improve your
mental frame of mind and ability to relax. Like all changes, this
requires practice and includes the following steps:

- **Listen carefully to what you say to or about yourself,
  both out loud and silently.** Pay special attention to the
  things you say during times that are particularly difficult.
- **Work on changing each negative statement to a
  positive one** that reflects your potential, strengths, and
  capabilities. For example, negative statements such as "I'll
  never make enough milk" or "I can't pump all the time so
  why bother" become positive messages such as "My breasts

were designed to make milk" or "I can pump five times a day, and that is really good."

- **Rehearse these positive statements**, mentally or with another person, as a replacement of those old, habitual negative statements.
- **Practice these new statements in real situations.** This practice, along with time and patience, will help the new patterns of thinking become automatic.

Psychological techniques aren't going to improve every situation, but they can't hurt, and if they help, you'll be glad you tried. At the very least, you'll have done something that is good for your own well-being, and if baby benefits, too, all the better!

Increasing Milk Production

Janelle's Story

I always had strangely shaped, tubular breasts, and during my first pregnancy, they never enlarged. At one week of age, my daughter Hannah was well under her birth weight, and we made an urgent call to a lactation consultant. We discovered that I didn't have a lot of milk-making breast tissue, even though my breasts were long. I did make milk, but only a little—just .25 ounces (10 milliliters) per feeding. I started pumping immediately, along with goat's rue and More Milk Plus™ tincture every feeding. Every two hours I nursed Hannah on each side, pumped for ten minutes, fed her what I'd pumped, and then finished with formula. Gradually, my milk production increased. Soon, I had enough milk to make it through night feedings with just me! At two months, because I breastfed very often and Hannah nursed willingly, we decided to stop pumping but maintain the herbs. By three months, I was down to two evening bottles, and at age four months, Hannah decided not to take a supplemental bottle at all. She continued to gain weight at the same pace and was a healthy baby. The work was hard, but the rewards were great!

With my second baby, I had high hope that things would kick in right away, but again my breasts didn't grow, and my milk did not come in. I was so crushed, but I knew there was light at the end of the tunnel. I started pumping and taking the herbs, eventually trading domperidone for the More Milk Plus. It wasn't long before my milk supply was over the top and able to fill her little belly. Would I do it the same way all over again? You bet! I feel so fulfilled as a mother of two breastfed infants.

CHAPTER 11

Physical Techniques to Make More Milk

Now it's time to explore options for increasing your supply. Start with ideas that most closely address the root of your problem. *Targeting your treatment to the causes you've identified will increase your odds for improvement.* Physical techniques are the first line of defense when attempting to increase milk production because they capitalize on the principle of "demand and supply." In uncomplicated cases of low milk production, it can take two to three days to notice a change. Results for more complicated cases may take longer, depending on the underlying cause. Physical techniques are often effective by themselves, or they can be combined with other techniques.

Breastfeed More Frequently

Not breastfeeding often enough is the number one cause of low milk production and the easiest to reverse. How often has your baby been nursing in a twenty-four-hour day? Especially in the first few weeks, mothers with vulnerable supplies shouldn't allow longer than two to three hours between daytime feedings or longer than one four- to five-hour sleep stretch each day. It's normal for a newborn to nurse *at least* eight times in twenty-four hours, and when milk production is low, feeding more often than this is baby's way of telling the breast that he needs more milk. If you don't change anything, the breast won't change what it's doing, either. Would your baby nurse more often if you offered? The simple solution is to offer.

One way to encourage more frequent breastfeeding is to take a "babymoon" vacation at home with baby. Spend the weekend in bed together, cuddling and nursing. Take magazines, snacks, and beverages with you, and read, nap, knit, talk on the phone, or watch television. This vacation will not only help to encourage frequent nursing, but it will also result in a better-rested baby and mother, and likely more milk by Monday.

Breast Massage and Compressions

Massage helps bring milk forward for easy removal and also helps stimulate milk ejection, which may be weaker with lower milk volume. Work from your chest forward toward your nipple with kneading or circular hand movements, using comfortable pressure. But don't limit it to feeding time. Breast massage for general stimulation and enhancement is practiced in some cultures and is one of those "can't hurt, may help" ideas.

Breast compressions (described in Chapter 5) enhance milk removal by adding pressure inside the breast to propel milk through the ducts for easier removal by baby or pump. Start compressing when baby's swallowing slows or when the flow slows for the pump; stop when swallowing or flow stops and repeat until it isn't helping anymore. This easy and effective technique should be a part of every low-milk-supply strategy.

Warmth

Warm, moist compresses applied to the breasts just prior to nursing or pumping can also help the milk to start flowing. There are commercial products, but you can make your own by filling a sock with uncooked non-instant rice and tying the end closed.

The shape of the sock allows it to be wrapped comfortably around your breasts. Lightly dampen it and microwave for about thirty seconds so the sock is warm but not hot. A warm, wet washcloth is also helpful. Hot showers are famous for initiating milk ejection, although they may not always be convenient. You can even try nursing your baby in a warm bath.

Touch

Any form of nipple stimulation, such as gentle tickling, rolling, or pulling, can encourage milk ejection when you're feeling stressed or anxious. Reverse pressure softening, often used for engorgement, is an easy and effective variation. Read more about this technique at www.kellymom.com/bf/concerns/mom/ rev_pressure_soft_cotterman.html.

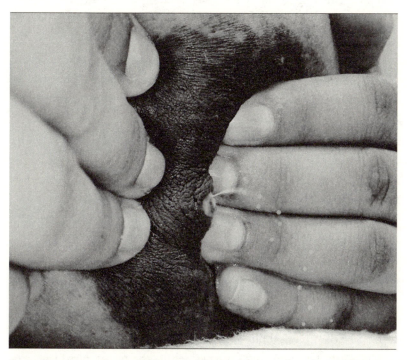

Reverse pressure softening (RPS) can help soften a firm areola and stimulate milk ejection.

Shoulder massages and back rubs also seem to have an effect on the reflex. One particularly effective method is to have someone "spine walk" their knuckles on either side of your spine, from neck to waist. This may cause a shiver or chill sensation that also triggers milk ejection. Another technique is to have someone massage your shoulder close to the neck as you're nursing or pumping to stimulate an acupressure point that can trigger milk ejection. At the very least, you'll feel relaxed after this "spa" treatment!

Pumping

Pumping, commonly recommended first to increase milk production, can be an excellent tool, though it isn't always necessary. If your baby is nursing often *and effectively* and also enjoys comfort nursing, his sucking may be doing such a good job that extra pumping isn't needed. Supplementing at breast or supplementing first and finishing at the breast may be adequate. You may choose to pump even when baby nurses well to strengthen the "make more" message. But if your baby isn't nursing effectively or sucks only the short time that milk is flowing, pumping becomes the primary way to stimulate the breasts. The best strategy depends on your pumping goals. Are you trying to achieve a full milk supply or concentrating more on increasing your current supply? Will you pump for a few weeks to maximize your production capability, or longer if necessary?

Choosing a Breast Pump

There are many types of breast pumps available to nursing mothers, through both rental and purchase. *Hospital-grade* electric pumps are multiuser rental pumps built for both performance and endurance. All models are auto-cycling and have adjustable vacuum suction; some also have adjustable cycling speeds. They are usually rented rather than purchased because they are expensive (US$700 to US$1,500). Rental rates are more affordable (US$40 to US$80 per month). The personal kit to attach to the pump motor is purchased separately and must match the pump brand; *they are not interchangeable.* The two major pump manufacturers of hospital-grade and higher-end consumer-grade pumps are Ameda (www .ameda.com) and Medela (www.medela.com, which also carries scales).

Consumer-grade electric pumps are usually single-user and range from highly effective pumps that can last one or more years under heavy use to light-duty pumps intended for use a few times a week. The higher-end pumps can handle dual pumping at full suction. Lighter-duty pumps have lower suction with the dual pumping setting. All dual pumps may seem capable of the same performance, *but they are not.*

To be effective, a good pump balances both suction strength and cycling speed to approximate the sucking of a baby. Pumps that reach their pressure too quickly cause tissue damage, as can those that take too much time to build up to the appropriate pressure. Some high-end consumer-grade pumps claim to have similar specifications to hospital-grade pumps but differ in their endurance and longevity. Mothers almost universally find that they are able to extract milk more easily and quickly with hospital-grade pumps than with even the best consumer-grade pumps.

As tempting as it may be to cut corners, it is important to remember that smaller, cheaper pumps wear out quickly and don't draw milk as efficiently. Check the warranty for the expected life of any pump you're considering. Your breast pump is an investment in you and your baby and should be the best tool you can afford. If you can't afford a good electric pump, a good manual pump is often more effective than a poor-quality, inexpensive electric or battery-operated pump. Manual double pumping is possible with Medela's Lactina kit if your arm is long enough to hold both flanges and have a free hand to pull the piston. The kit also can be attached to their foot-driven pedal pump.

Breast flanges, or "breast shields," are the funnel-shaped parts that fit against the breast. Medela and Ameda offer multiple flange sizes to improve the comfort and effectiveness of a pump. Proper fit is critical to effective milk removal. A flange that is too small can cause friction, soreness, or nipple swelling. A flange that is too large may pull in too much tissue, causing swelling and redness. The average flange tunnel is 24 to 26 millimeters, but many women seem to do better with the next size up, which is 27 to 29 millimeters. To know if the flange you're using fits well, watch the way your nipple draws into the flange tunnel as you pump. It's normal to touch the sides of the tunnel, but it should move easily. Your areola should move slightly, as well. A small amount of olive oil can lubricate the tunnel and alleviate friction, but a properly sized flange shouldn't need it. Any marks or redness on the areola or at the nipple base after pumping are signs that the flange doesn't fit. Try the next larger size. If larger doesn't feel better, try smaller. Softer, more flexible silicone flanges are available, though they may come in only one size.

Hand Expression

Expressing by hand is the oldest method of extracting milk and can be an effective way to increase production. Hand expression is an art that comes naturally to some women but is more difficult to learn for others. It should be done for as long and as often as you would use a mechanical pump. Expressing into a soft plastic cup or bowl lets you aim into a large container that can be squeezed for pouring. For pictures and an explanation of the technique, see

Used Pumps

It's common to see pumps at yard sales and online resale sites like eBay. They may also be handed down from a friend or sister. If it's hospital-grade, there's a good chance that it was stolen at some point. Ask for the serial number and contact the rental company, who will tell you for sure. Used consumer-grade models abound but can be contaminated with bacteria, mold, and viruses or simply be worn down from use so they no longer draw milk out well as they once did. Your supply is vulnerable; why take a chance and waste your hard work by using a pump that no longer performs well?

www.nursingmother.com/helpme/helpme_images_expression
.html.

Pumping Techniques

Simultaneously pumping both breasts is usually the fastest and most effective way to remove milk and may stimulate a higher prolactin surge.[1] Hold each bottle or flange with a separate hand or use one arm to reach around to the opposite breast while tucking the first bottle against the breast with the inside of the same arm, leaving one hand free. There are bras and straps that can hold the pump flanges to allow hands-free pumping, or you can create your own by cutting small slits in a snug sports bra. Single pumping may be more comfortable if you make a lot more on one side than the other. This allows you to alternate breasts while pumping, which sometimes yields more milk. Single pumping definitely makes it easier to do breast compressions on the breast that is being pumped.

As with nursing, it's important to be comfortable while pumping. Many mothers jam the flanges deep into their breasts, elbows sticking out and their backs curled over so they can watch the milk come out or because they've been told they have to lean over to pump. No wonder some say it's a miserable experience! Instead, find a comfortable spot with supportive pillows so you can lean back. The amount of milk pumped doesn't increase with leaning forward, so you may as well be comfortable. One caveat: the milk may stay in the flange tunnel because of the angle and can leak back onto the breast if you don't rock forward periodically to empty it into the bottle. One option if this is a real problem for you are Pumpin' Pal International's Super Shields, tilted flanges that fit into your flanges so that the milk flows forward when you are leaning back, eliminating leakage.

Pumping Strategies

Pumping requires patience, persistence, and a consistent, workable plan, but there is no one right way to go about it. The best way to pump is the way that works for you—flexibility is the key. If you struggle with pumping every feeding, then maybe a goal of pumping every other feeding is more realistic and attainable. Occasionally, you might even breastfeed one feeding and pump the next. Figure out what you *can* do and start with that so that you can feel good about it rather than guilty for what didn't happen.

Pump After Feeds. The most common approach to increasing supply by pumping is to nurse as long as baby will actively suck, and then pump. This is especially appropriate when baby is leaving a lot of milk in the breast, but also for the baby who sucks well only the short time that milk is flowing strongly. Whatever residual milk the pump removes then becomes baby's next supplement before any formula. Pump until the milk stops, but at least ten to twenty minutes (the shorter the feed, the longer the pumping time), even if there is no milk flowing during some of this time. Don't stop just because the milk seems to have stopped. *The amount of milk you pump does not matter* because baby should be taking the majority of it first. Your goal is extra stimulation to tell your body to make more milk than it is making right now. If baby tends to nurse actively for a short while but then spends a lot of time mostly hanging out, limit his time on the breast to active suckling—even if that's only five minutes per side—so that you have enough time to supplement him, pump, and keep your sanity.

Pump Between Feeds. If seeing only a little milk is discouraging, pumping between feedings or halfway through a nap rather than right after can provide that visible feedback you want. It also may become more of an extra session rather than the continuation of your feeding session as far as your body is concerned. At the least, having more milk to remove means more for your body to replace. The downside is that there may be less milk in the breast for baby if he wakes up too soon.

Pump During the Night. If you can handle it, pumping at night takes advantage of any higher prolactin levels in addition to removing more milk. However, getting adequate sleep is also important to your overall health and well-being and can affect your milk production. The trick is to be flexible in balancing the two. Try to plan for at least one pumping session in the middle of the night if you can. Or don't set an alarm, but if you happen to awaken, use that opportunity. The sedating effects of oxytocin being released while pumping may help you get back to sleep when you're done. Taking a couple of short naps in the daytime can help you stay rested.

Power Pumping. Catherine Watson Genna, B.S., IBCLC, suggests an alternative short-term strategy for mothers of healthy, full-term babies who are having a difficult time fitting pumping into their busy daytime routines. Place the breast pump in a convenient location that you will pass often and where you'll be comfortable sitting or standing. Every time you pass the pump, use it for five to ten minutes or so, as often as every forty-five to sixty minutes. Stop when you begin to feel "antsy," restless, or annoyed. You can continue pumping into the same bottle and pumping kit for four to six hours without refrigeration, depending on the temperature in the room. After four to six hours, take the accumulated milk to the refrigerator, wash the kit, and start fresh for the next four to six hours. Aim for pumping at least ten times every day. Continue for two to three days and then resume your normal pumping routine.

Taking a Break from the Hamster Wheel. Pumping can be a lot of work! The never-ending cycles of supplementing, breastfeeding, and pumping can become exhausting and overwhelming and sometimes seem impossible, especially if you have older children who also need attention. You might wonder if you should just give up. What you probably need is a break, and it's absolutely fine to take one. Jan Ellen Brown, RDH, IBCLC, works with many mothers who feel like they're on this "hamster wheel." She recommends simplifying the routine by just pumping for two or three days (be sure to do it at least eight to ten times a day!) and feed-

What If Baby Cries When You're Pumping?

Your baby's emotional needs come first, and nothing is as important as comforting him. You can always resume pumping later, or even just skip until the next time. Pumping should never cause you or your baby emotional stress.

ing baby that milk by an alternate method. This strategy not only gives you a few days off to catch your breath but also can result in increased milk from thorough, consistent milk removal. When you're feeling better, add breastfeeding back in. Most babies don't have difficulty coming back to breast after such a short time when using the alternative feeding techniques described in Chapter 4, especially bottle-feeding methods that support breastfeeding.

How Long Do I Keep This Up?

Once you've reached your goal, baby can often keep your supply going and you can stop pumping. Congratulations—you're done! But what if you need the pump to keep supply up? Or maybe you've hit a ceiling and find you aren't getting any more milk no matter what you do. If you've been pumping very often, try reducing the frequency and see if your body maintains your production level. If so, great! Should production drop just a little, decide if it's worth the extra effort to maintain the higher level. A small number of women find that they actually get *more* milk when they back off. Ultimately you'll want to use the pump as little as you can get away with. Experimentation will help you find the balance where you get the most milk for your work.

Alternative Therapies

Alternative therapies such as chiropractics, acupuncture, acupressure, and yoga are attractive options because they use only external techniques to stimulate milk supply or milk release. They have the most potential for mothers with normal mammary tissue.

Chiropractics

Chiropractics focus on the neurological effects of spinal joint dysfunction. Somewhat accidentally, it has been discovered that chiropractic adjustments sometimes can help increase milk production in women whose spinal vertebrae move out of position and compress or irritate spinal nerves, which is known as *subluxation*. Three cases were recently described in a chiropractic journal. While all the mothers had low milk supply, only one was seeking help for that specifically. It was her second baby, and she had made plenty of milk for her first. The second mother had back pain, while the third thought her baby's suck was the problem and so wanted help for her baby. Problems were identified with the first two women for treatment. In the third case, the doctor found nothing wrong with the baby's suck, so she examined the mother and found several vertebral problems. Each case was very different in history and problems, but within the first few treatments, milk supply increased and eventually reached 100 percent.[2] Chiropractic treatment may work by restoring nerve communication in key areas that have been reduced or cut off. This approach may be worth investigating when there is no other explanation but there is a history of physical trauma, nerve pain, numbness, or impingements.

Acupuncture and Acupressure

Acupuncture is a traditional Chinese medicine (TCM) therapeutic practice during which specific areas on the body are pierced with very fine needles. *Acupressure*, also called *shiatsu*, is the application of pressure with thumbs or fingertips to points on the body for therapeutic effects, while *reflexology* focuses on trigger points in the foot. Although not as common in the Western world, acupuncture in particular has been used to treat low milk production for over two thousand years. Research conducted in multiple countries suggests that it can be effective. Acupuncture can stimulate both prolactin and oxytocin, depending on the points chosen by the practitioner. Because TCM relies on a thorough screening of the patient to select the proper treatment locations, mothers interested in acupuncture or acupressure treatments for low milk production should seek an experienced and qualified practitioner, who may teach techniques that can be used at home as well. Acupuncture may not be as effective for low production when there is poor breast development.[3]

Yoga

Yoga is a system of exercises to promote control of the body and mind. Awtar Kaur Khalsa, M.A., IBCLC, RYT, a registered yoga teacher and International Board Certified Lactation Consultant, reports that several lactating yoga students experienced increases in milk volume after attending her Kundalini yoga classes. She believes that arm movements increase blood circulation, which in turn causes relaxation and easier milk flow. Other mothers have reported increases after various upper arm activities, supporting the idea that such movements can stimulate milk production. From a practical standpoint, yoga is an effective means of exercise and relaxation that is safe for pregnant and breastfeeding mothers. At the very least, the relaxation it affords can help facilitate milk ejection.

CHAPTER 12

Galactogogues: Foods, Herbs, and Medications That Stimulate Milk Production

Throughout time, in every country and culture, mothers have taken special foods or herbs to help them make milk. We don't have nearly enough scientific documentation yet to prove their effectiveness, but many of these traditions are supported by centuries of experience. Cultural wisdom, though not always proven accurate, often contains truth that is worth considering.

If you bypassed earlier chapters and skipped to this one looking for an immediate way to increase supply, keep in mind that galactogogues can't compensate for a milk supply problem if milk removal is not sufficiently frequent and effective. Identifying and addressing all contributing factors to your low production first will give you the best shot at success. *Then*, galactogogues may help speed up the process.

The decision of when to use galactogogues should be made based on your circumstances and personal comfort level and with the input of your lactation counselors and/or health care providers. In most cases, it's wise to give your body at least four to seven days after birth to try and do its job before intervening. Prolactin-stimulating drugs and herbs are less likely to be effective until prolactin begins to drop toward the end of the first or second week (unless you know you have low prolactin). It usually takes at least four to seven days to see the initial galactogogue effect, though some response may be seen within forty-eight hours. Simple situations involving secondary causes usually require only short-term use, approximately one to four weeks. Once full milk production is reestablished, the galactogogue is gradually reduced. In more difficult cases, a galactogogue may be required indefinitely to sustain a higher level of milk production, though many mothers find that they can reduce their dosages after the first six months.

Targeting: Choosing the Best Galactogogue for Your Needs

The most common Western strategy is to boost prolactin, typically with prolactin-stimulating medications. As discussed in Chapter 1, prolactin is high at birth to get milk production started but then normally decreases to moderately elevated levels as milk removal takes over driving milk production. However, extra prolactin (brought about by galactogogues or physical stimulation) can boost milk production further in many women. And it can inhibit or even reverse the process of mammary involution—the tearing down of your milk factory—that might otherwise start when production has slowed down.[1] This helps sustain your milk-making cells, which is especially important when there are fewer due to hypoplasia or breast surgery. Extra prolactin can also compensate for mild deficiencies of some hormones.[2]

Though boosting prolactin can be effective for many mothers, it doesn't bring the best results for everyone. Just as there is no one best antibiotic to treat every infection, there is no one substance that can increase milk production best in all situations. When selecting a drug, herb, or food to help with your milk production, consider which have other properties that are helpful for your situation, such as an antiandrogen herbal galactogogue if you have excessive testosterone or a high-iron herb if you are anemic. *Targeting your choice to your situation may improve your chances of increasing milk production.*

Pharmaceutical Galactogogues

There are no pharmaceutical drugs that have been specifically designated by the U.S. Food and Drug Administration (FDA) as galactogogues to date. Several drugs that are marketed for other disorders do, however, have the side effect of increasing milk production; such "off-label" use is a legitimate practice. Some people believe that pharmaceutical galactogogues are more effective than herbal ones, but others report better results from herbs. The differences in opinion may be due to how appropriately each one addressed the mother's underlying problem, or due to varying dosages or potencies.

Domperidone (Motilium™)

Domperidone is a prescription antinausea and stomach-emptying drug that is used for gastrointestinal disorders in adults and children. It also increases prolactin and can have a dramatic effect on milk production.[3] Because domperidone has an excellent safety profile, it is considered the drug of choice for increasing milk production where it is available.[4] Many physicians have prescribed domperidone over the years to improve lactation and report excellent results in general with very few side effects, though it can't completely compensate for insufficient glandular tissue. The American Academy of Pediatrics rates domperidone as "usually compatible with breastfeeding," and Dr. Thomas Hale rates it L1 (safest) in *Medications and Mothers' Milk*.

The most accepted galactogogue dosage of domperidone in North America is 10 to 30 milligrams three to four times a day for a total of 30 to 90 milligrams daily.[5] A recent Australian study tested both infant safety and the dosage response of 30 and 60 milligrams (the common dosage range) of domperidone for one week each in six mothers with preterm babies and low milk supply. Four of the mothers had significant increases in milk production with just 30 milligrams of domperidone, and three of those four mothers had further increases at 60 milligrams. No other milk supply risk factors besides preterm delivery were taken into account. The amount the babies received through the milk was extremely low, less than 1 percent, reaffirming the safety of domperidone during lactation.[6]

Interestingly, some mothers have needed as much as 120 milligrams per day to maximize their supplies. It may be that the underlying cause of low milk production, rarely addressed in studies, affects some mothers' responsiveness to domperidone and so requires a higher dosage for significant results. This needs to be researched further. A recent study of use for gastrointestinal problems showed "excellent safety" in doses of 120 milligrams, and diabetic patients with digestion problems have used up to 120 milligrams daily for as long as twelve years without ill effects.[7] Until there is more research, that's the maximum dose experts consider to be safe for increasing milk production. However, the ramifications of long-term use in breastfeeding mothers and babies haven't been studied.

More detailed information on domperidone as a galactogogue exists than for other medications because so many mothers have taken it and shared their experiences. It is well tolerated in almost all circumstances, and the only known caution is for mothers who have a prolonged QTc interval, a particular type of heart problem. A few women may experience abdominal cramping, dry mouth, or headaches.[8] Women on the higher dosages have reported increased appetites and weight gain that reverse when they stop taking it; one mother found that the addition of fennel helped to curb her appetite. A few mothers also reported feeling blue when they cut down quickly, so be sure to wean down gradually over several weeks.

Domperidone is considered to be safe and effective by the regulatory agencies of the European countries and is available without prescription in many countries, including Ireland, Italy, Netherlands, China, South Africa, Mexico, New Zealand, and Chile. However, its use for increasing milk production has become controversial in the United States, where it has not been through the FDA review process because competing drugs already available don't make it worth the expensive process. For this reason, it is not available from standard U.S. pharmacies, though some compounding pharmacies will make it by prescription. For further information and updates on the status of domperidone in the United States, consult our website, www.lowmilksupply.org/domperidone.shtml.

Metoclopramide (Reglan™, Maxeran™)

Metoclopramide is commonly used to treat gastroesophageal reflux in both adults and children. Since it increases prolactin and can stimulate milk production by 66 to 100 percent, metoclopramide has been used unofficially to increase milk production for nearly three decades.[9] However, unlike domperidone, it crosses the blood-brain barrier and can cause central nervous system side effects such as restlessness, drowsiness, fatigue, depression, and involuntary body movements, especially when used longer than two to four weeks.[10] These problems are considered uncommon when taken for gastrointestinal problems, but postpartum women seem to be more vulnerable, and complaints of fatigue and blueness are common. It also may not be compatible with selective serotonin reuptake inhibitor (SSRI) antidepressants.[11] If you have a personal or family history of depression, it's probably wise to avoid using metoclopramide. The most common effective dose is 10 to 15 milligrams three times per day *for no longer than three weeks.*[12] The American Academy of Pediatrics considers it a "drug whose effect on nursing infants is unknown but may be of concern," while Hale rates it L2 (safer).

Metformin (Glucophage™)

Metformin is an insulin receptor–sensitizing agent used for type 2 diabetes and often for polycystic ovary syndrome (PCOS) as well.

171

Its predecessor, phenformin, was originally derived from galegin in the herb goat's rue. Metformin improves milk production for some PCOS mothers in a way that is not yet completely understood.[13] It also is considered compatible with breastfeeding and is rated L1 (safest) by Hale.

Since lactation is a new and experimental use of the drug, a prudent starting dose is the amount that was most effective if you were previously taking it. Metformin can cause diarrhea and stomach upset, so it should be started slowly, increasing gradually to an effective amount. Typical dosages range from 500 to 2,500 milligrams per day, but informal reports of success for lactation seem to occur in the 1,500 to 2,500 milligram range.

Metformin is more likely to work when there is a decent amount of mammary tissue; it can't compensate for hypoplasia. Infertility specialist Dr. Randall Craig reports that mothers in his practice who needed metformin for conception and stayed on it throughout pregnancy and into lactation seem to have better overall glandular development and milk production.

Lactogenic Foods: Setting the Stage for a Good Milk Supply

Traditional societies view food as more than just nutrition; it is also their medicine. New mothers are fed foods believed to support good milk production, and special concoctions may be created if more milk is needed. In the East Indian Ayurvedic tradition, almonds, coconut, and sesame seeds are considered to promote "rich" milk, while rice pudding with milk and sugar, pumpkin, sunflower seeds, and sesame seeds are often recommended to support or increase production.[14] In the Chinese tradition, foods that are considered supportive of lactation strengthen the center and regulate body warmth and fluids. These include chicken (with bones) and seaweed soups, cooked (usually green) papaya, millet, rice, anise, fennel, dill, cumin, caraway, and ginger. Other foods reputed to be lactogenic include lettuce, prickly lettuce, champignon mushrooms, barley, oats, chickpeas, dandelion, and pounded rice cakes. Many have nutrients that probably play a role in their reputation. Some, like sesame seeds, are high in calcium, while others are high in omega-3 fatty acids, vitamins, minerals, or iron.

Grain-based beverages are popular in many traditional cultures to help new mothers develop a strong milk supply. *Atole* is a popular Mexican beverage made with oats or cornmeal simmered in milk. Barley water, made with ½ cup of flaked or pearled barley simmered in 1 quart (946 milliliters) of water for twenty minutes, especially with added fennel seed, is an Old-World remedy. In European countries, commercial coffee-substitute beverages made from roasted grains (Cafix, Pero, Kaffree Roma, and Dandy Blend) are popular for increasing milk production; their common ingredient is barley. Oatmeal is popular with North American nursing mothers. Steel-cut or rolled oats are more nutritious and likely to be more effective than instant. Oats are also high in fiber, as is brown rice and most other whole grains and dried beans. See www.mother-food.com and www.mobimotherhood.org for recipes and more information.

Navigating the World of Herbal Galactogogues

While herbal galactogogues have been used for centuries in traditional cultures, Western mothers are turning to them more than ever in their desperate search for answers. The information that follows will help you decide if they are right for you, which are most appropriate, and what to consider in looking for a quality product.

Effectiveness of Herbal Galactogogues

Our basic knowledge about herbs comes from four major sources: the German Commission E monographs (a compilation of expert herbal reviews), ethnobotanical studies, herbal practitioners/researchers, and oral and written tradition about these herbs (including informal reports). Research is the gold standard for judging the effectiveness and safety of a substance, but the little herbal research that does exist is not the best. One major concern is the reliability of laboratory analysis. Researchers often break plants down to their individual nutritional and chemical components and then comment on the relative action or safety of each of these components *without regard for how they function together*. Laboratory analysis is limited in its ability to analyze the whole plant, where the balance of the combined parts may actually be safer than individual parts. The same is true for animal research, which provides insights but cannot automatically be applied to humans. Not all mammals react equally to various plants, and a plant that is dangerous for one can be safe for another.

Herbs can't rival the precision of manufactured drugs. Coming from plants, they are inherently variable and can be contaminated with other herbs or medications. Different parts of a plant can have different effects, and the timing of harvest and the method of preservation and preparation can affect the useful properties. Herbs have limited shelf lives, and time and light exposure affect their potency. Because of this, effectiveness can vary by brand, crop, and batch.

The guidance of trained practitioners is invaluable. *Herbalists* have training from lore passed down from one generation to the next, formal or self-education, research, or apprenticeship. *Doctors of traditional Chinese medicine* (TCM) are formally trained to use herbs based on a thousand-year-old tradition, while *naturopaths*, doctors whose specialty includes the use of botanical medicine, are familiar with both modern medicine and traditional herbal medicine and represent a blending of Eastern and Western thought.

Most herbs have multiple properties or actions within the body. Many that are used as galactogogues also help digestion or bring on the flow of menses, and a few may stimulate prolactin, though unfortunately research has rarely looked at this. Some, including those reputed to increase breast size, contain phytoestrogens and so are considered "estrogenic," though they do not act the same as estrogen. Recommendations that herbs with phytoestrogens should not be used in lactation are based on the theoretical concern that phytoestrogens will suppress milk production in the same way as natural estrogen. This has not been borne out of real-life experience, and in fact, phytoestrogens are considered by herb experts to stimulate mammary growth and support lactation.

Tell baby's and your health care providers whenever you use herbs to increase milk production. When used in larger amounts, some herbs can interact negatively with some drugs or cause side effects, such as diarrhea or a maple-syrup-scented urine, that might be misinterpreted if the doctor doesn't know about them.

Safety of Herbal Galactogogues

Toxicology studies have shown the more widely available herbs to be relatively safe, although most of the formal research is with dairy animals.[15] Be aware of the safety of your herb source; some imported from Asia can be contaminated with heavy metals.[16]

A question frequently asked is whether an herb will get into the milk and if that is a problem. There isn't much research, but it's reasonable to apply the same principles as for medications used while nursing, which have an average transfer rate of about 1 percent. As with medications, transference into the milk is rarely an issue for baby. An excellent resource is Sheila Humphrey's book *The Nursing Mother's Herbal*, which rates a long list of commonly used herbs according to their relative safety for nursing.

Herbs Come in Many Forms

If you stroll down the aisle of your local drug or health food store, you'll quickly notice that herbs come in a variety of forms. There are whole-herb preparations that grind up all the usable parts and package them as powders, tablets, or capsules, and there are "standardized extracts" that guarantee a certain amount of active ingredients from the herb for a standard dose. Tinctures extract certain plant properties by soaking the herb in alcohol or another medium at various concentrations, while teas steep dried leaves, flowers, seeds, or roots in hot water to extract their water-soluble properties.

Which form is best? Not even the experts agree, as they each have their own philosophy, and the method of preparation plays a strong role in the herbs' effectiveness. For instance, the medicinal properties in tea that isn't given enough brewing time won't be as strong; if it is brewed too long, it may become very bitter. Some herbs in tablet form have a small proportion of active ingredients, while others are quite potent. The right form, in most cases, is probably the one you like best, though in some cases form is important, and women often find that one works better for them than another.

How to Take Galactogogues

Some herbs and medications should not be taken together. For instance, those that contain a lot of fiber (typically dried herbs/seeds, loose or in capsules) can slow the absorption of some medications. It is important to research your other prescription medications for any documented interactions with herbs. *The PDR for Herbal Medicines*, edited by Joerg Gruenwald, Thomas Brendler, and Christof Jaenicke (Thomson Healthcare, 2007), is a reputable resource.

Sweeteners can be added to bitter teas, or tinctures can be mixed with a *small* amount of strong juice or tea to mask the flavors (larger amounts might diminish its effectiveness). However, some herbalists believe that it is necessary to experience the bitter flavor in order to stimulate gastric juices sufficiently for full absorption into the bloodstream. Foods taken at the same time as herbs may aid or interfere with absorption, depending on the individual qualities of the herb. For this reason, it's important to pay attention to instructions regarding when and how to take each herb. Consider taking herbs and medications at different times as well.

You may also find that rotating galactogogue herbs every few weeks, as suggested by some authors, allows fresh stimulation and prevents the body from becoming used to a substance and responding less over time.[17]

Herbal Dosages

One of the challenges in using herbs as galactogogues is the dearth of information on therapeutic dosage amounts. With the exception of a few herbs like blessed thistle and fenugreek, most of the recommendations for dosages are quite standard. Yet, in most cases, there are no studies to see if these amounts are adequate for increasing milk production or if the amounts needed might vary according to the underlying problem.

Some herbs are completely benign and can be experimented with freely, while others may be potentially toxic in large amounts and must be used much more carefully. Start with the basic recommended dosages. Primary problems may take much longer to respond than simple management or baby-related problems. *Titration*, the upward or downward adjustment of a dose to meet the need, is often necessary. The concept of "if a little is good, more is better" is *not* true for all herbal galactogogues. When you find something effective, use no more than is necessary, and when you want to cut back, do so gradually to help the body begin "taking back" its own duties. Allow at least a week between changes so long as you aren't experiencing any negative side effects.

Targeting Herbs to the Cause of the Problem

You may be wondering where to start in choosing herbs. Alfalfa, fenugreek, goat's rue, nettle, and shatavari are good all-purpose galactogogues that usually work well for low milk supply due to secondary causes. If you prefer familiar cooking herbs, try eating or making a tea from crushed anise, caraway, coriander, dill, or fennel seed. But if you have specific issues related to your low supply, look more closely for herbs with additional properties that may address your problem. The appendix includes a summary of herbal properties most likely to help low production.

Galactogogue Herbs

The following is an overview of key herbs reputed to help with milk production. Refer to the appendix for starting dosage information.

Alfalfa (*Medicago Sativa*). A popular, nutritious, and commonly used galactogogue, alfalfa is often taken in combination with blessed thistle, marshmallow, and fenugreek. It should be avoided if you have lupus or another autoimmune disorder as alfalfa seeds and sprouts, including tablets, contain L-canavanine, which has been found to cause or exacerbate lupus symptoms.[18]

Aniseed or Anise Seed (*Pimpinella Anisum*). One of the "aromatic" herbs and a traditional medicine in France, anise seed is known for helping colic and gassiness as well as increasing milk production. It is considered to be mildly estrogenic, and some believe it may help with milk ejection. It is *not* the same as *star of anise* and should not be used interchangeably.

Blessed Thistle (*Cnicus Benedictus*). The use of blessed thistle has been recorded as far back as the early sixteenth century for treating many ailments and is considered to be a hormone balancer. It is a popular galactogogue that is most often taken in conjunction with fenugreek. Most mothers prefer to take blessed thistle in capsule form as the teas and tinctures are quite bitter.

Borage (*Borago Officinalis*). A lesser-known lactogenic herb, borage also has a reputation for helping with premenstrual syndrome, endometriosis, and fibrocystic breasts. Its leaves contain small amounts of toxic alkaloids, making it somewhat controversial for use by breastfeeding mothers despite its ability to increase milk production. Borage *oil* is made from borage seeds and contains very little of these alkaloids, so it can be safely consumed when used appropriately.[19] High in the beneficial fat gamma-linolenic acid (GLA), it also has the reputation of increasing the creaminess of the milk.

Caraway Seed (*Carum Carvi*). Another of the aromatic galactogogue herbs, caraway is also known for its anticolic and antiflatulence properties. It has a reputation for increasing the flow of milk in nursing mothers. Caraway also is often combined with other galactogogue herbs.

Chasteberry, Chaste Tree Berry, or Vitex (*Vitex Agnus-Castus*).
The chaste tree berry derived its name for maintaining chastity
among monks. It is well known for its normalizing effects on the
pituitary gland and especially on progesterone (probably by helping ovulation) and is believed to regulate prolactin. It is often
taken for premenstrual syndrome, irregular menstruation, infertility, and even acne.

Chasteberry has long had a reputation for increasing milk production, and some believe it may also aid milk ejection. As far
back as A.D. 50, Dioscorides recommended chaste tree fruit for
"stimulating milk flow in nursing mothers." Research conducted
in the early 1940s and 1953 showed that mothers who took chasteberry experienced increases of up to 80 percent and "freer flow" of
milk.[20] Herb expert David Hoffman notes that chasteberry "can be
safely taken throughout the end of the third month of pregnancy
. . . which may prevent miscarriage" but is not recommended after
that "because it may bring on the flow of milk too early."[21]

Confusingly, recent research has documented decreases in prolactin, calling into question chasteberry's use as a galactogogue.
Studies in men show that low doses of chasteberry (120 milligrams
per day) stimulate prolactin, while high doses (500 milligrams per
day) lower it. Rats injected with large amounts showed apparent decreases in milk production. This has caused many to shelve
chasteberry as a galactogogue, though the issue of dosage may
hold the key. Chasteberry is probably not a good choice as a general galactogogue but may be appropriate if hormonal imbalances
are part of your milk production problem.

Dandelion (*Taraxacum Officinale*). Dandelion leaves (yes, those
weeds in the lawn!) are considered to be lactogenic and good
to use when milk is slow to come in and you have postpartum
edema. Potassium contributes to its diuretic properties. Dandelion
is also considered antidiabetic. It can be taken as a tincture or tea,
or young dandelion leaves not treated with chemicals can be eaten
in a salad or cooked.

Dill Seed (*Anethum Graveolens*). Widely used since ancient times for digestive issues, dill seed is part of the recipe for "gripe water," traditionally used to soothe infant colic. It is included in many popular commercial galactogogue products because it seems to work especially well when combined with other galactogogues. Dill seed is also one of the herbs thought to facilitate milk ejection; herb expert David Hoffman states that it "will stimulate the flow of milk in nursing mothers."[22] It can be sprinkled on food or taken as a tea.

Fennel (*Foeniculum Vulgare*). A popular European galactogogue, fennel is also known for its ability to reduce intestinal gas and improve digestion. Mothers of colicky babies may take fennel tea to simultaneously help their milk production and possibly calm baby's digestive upsets. Fennel is also reputed to be diuretic and antiandrogenic, may promote milk ejection, and has been studied for its ability to reduce inappropriate hair growth in women.[23] Its phytoestrogens likely play a role in its breast-enhancing reputation. Additionally, fennel may have appetite-suppressing properties; one mother reported that it helped mitigate her hunger while taking domperidone.

Fenugreek Seed (*Trigonella Foenum-Graecum*). Enjoyed in all parts of the world as a culinary herb, fenugreek lends its distinct flavor to a wide variety of baked goods and foods, including curry and imitation maple syrup. It is known to be quite nutritious, containing protein, iron, vitamin C, niacin, and potassium. Fenugreek is probably the most popular galactogogue herb among women in North America and is recommended frequently by lactation professionals. It is one of the oldest documented medicinal herbs and has been used as a galactogogue for both human mothers and dairy cows throughout the world. In one small study of humans, average milk output doubled.[24]

Animal research may be providing clues regarding the specific mechanism for increasing milk production. A study of buffaloes determined that fenugreek raised prolactin plasma levels, while another with goats concluded that growth hormone was stimulated.

Three to six grams per day (three capsules of the most commonly used size three times daily) is the most frequently recommended dosage.[25] If you have a sensitive stomach, start with a low dose and work up gradually. Your sweat and urine may smell like maple syrup when taking it. Allergic reactions to fenugreek are uncommon, but if you are prone to asthma or allergies, try a tincture rather than capsules. Fenugreek may not be a good choice if you have low thyroid because it lowered thyroid hormone (T3) in rats.[26]

Goat's Rue (*Galega Officinalis*). Native to southern Europe and western Asia, goat's rue was first mentioned in 1873 by dairy farmer Gillet-Damitte, who described milk production increases of between 35 to 50 percent in his cows when they were fed the plant.

Goat's rue comes from the same family as fenugreek and also has antidiabetic properties. It contains galegin, a guanidine compound from which the precursor to metformin was derived. Because metformin is beneficial in many cases of PCOS, goat's rue may be an especially appropriate galactogogue if you have PCOS. Goat's rue is also considered a diuretic and is reputed to increase breast tissue.

Despite the positive reports on cattle, toxic effects in sheep have made goat's rue somewhat controversial. The most plausible explanation for this is simply the variability of response in individual animals, though the grazing habits of sheep, who pull up and eat roots and all, has also been questioned. Goat's rue remains a popular galactogogue for French women and increasing numbers of North American women. We have not found any reports of human problems either anecdotally or in the literature. Herbalists who have clinical experience with goat's rue remain comfortable with its use.

Marshmallow Root (*Althaea Officinalis*). Although not actually a galactogogue itself, marshmallow root has a long anecdotal history of boosting the lactogenic effectiveness of fenugreek, blessed thistle, and alfalfa; some believe that it "enriches the milk" as well. It contains high levels of vitamin A, calcium, and zinc, as well as smaller amounts of iron, sodium, iodine, and B-complex vitamins. Combine marshmallow with other galactogogue herbs for maximum benefit.

Milk Thistle (*Silybum Marianum*). Milk thistle, sometimes called Mary's thistle, blessed milk thistle, or Lady's thistle, has been used medicinally for a wide range of liver and gall bladder problems since the first century in Europe. The fresh leaves can be eaten in salads or cooked as a spinach substitute. It is the favorite galactogogue of herb expert Dr. Tieraona Lowdog and is also used in traditional Chinese medicine. Capsules typically come in standardized form to guarantee the content of the active ingredient, silymarin.

Nettle or Stinging Nettle (*Urtica Urens* or *Urtica Dioica*). Nettle has also enjoyed a long tradition of medicinal use, dating back to ancient Greece. Rich in iron, calcium, vitamin K, and potassium, it is considered antidiabetic, diuretic, hypotensive, and supportive of thyroid function. It has a consistent history of being a powerful galactogogue and is a significant component of most commercial galactogogue products, though it is usually not used alone. The freeze-dried version of the herb, which is used in capsules and tinctures, is the most potent form. It is also the safest because leaves that have been dried in the usual fashion can contain mold spores, which could cause an allergic reaction in those sensitive to mold.

Oat Straw/Oats (*Avena Sativa*). Oat straw and its grain, oats, have enjoyed a long reputation as a galactogogue. Many different cultures use oats and oatmeal as foods for nursing mothers. Oats are very nutritious and easy to work into the diet: think oatmeal cereal, oatmeal cookies, oatmeal in breads, meat loaf, and *atole con avena*. Oat straw can also be found in capsules, tincture, and tea.

Red Clover Blossoms (*Trifolium Pratense*). As a galactogogue, red clover blossoms are usually combined with other herbs. They have multiple phytoestrogens to promote mammary development and also help to reduce edema. Ewes fed 3.5 kilograms of fermented red clover feed daily for two weeks had significantly increased total and free T3 thyroid hormone.[27] There is no information on whether normal doses of unfermented red clover affect thyroid hormone in humans, but it might be beneficial for mothers with low thyroid.

Red Raspberry (*Rubus Idaeus*). Red raspberry leaf is found in many galactogogue combination teas and tinctures, though it also is not considered a direct galactogogue. Its beneficial effects may be due to the nutritive value of the herb, and it may also aid milk ejection. The berries are considered to be helpful as well. Due to the astringent qualities of red raspberry, some herbalists believe that it may be useful in the short term but could cause a decrease in milk production if used long-term.[28] Red raspberry is usually combined with other galactogogues and may have a counteractive effect with those that cause loose stools.

Saw Palmetto (*Serenoa Repens*). Most known for its usefulness in treating male prostate conditions, saw palmetto is reported to have antiandrogenic and hormone balancing properties when used by women. Women who struggle with excessive body hair, male-pattern hair loss, or adult acne have turned to saw palmetto as a natural treatment for their problem.

Saw palmetto is often found in "natural" bust-enhancing products because of historic reports of breast enlargement with long-term use.[29] Herb expert David Hoffman notes that women with ovarian tenderness and enlargement or "small, undeveloped mammary glands" can benefit from saw palmetto and that "it increases the size and secreting power of the mammary glands where they are abnormally small and inactive."[30] The berries have also been used as galactogogues in animals, with reports of increased and richer milk in cows.[31] The use of saw palmetto in women in general has not been studied. In two cases of mothers with PCOS and low milk supply, saw palmetto was credited with increasing milk production when other herbs did not.

Shatavari (*Asparagus Racemosus*). From the Sanskrit, "she who has a hundred husbands," shatavari (or shatavri or shatawari) is known for its beneficial effects on women's reproductive function and is very popular as an all-around female tonic in India and China. It has traditionally been used for infertility problems and increasing milk production and is an ingredient in Lactare, an Indian commercial galactogogue product.

Shatavari increased the size of the mammary gland in rats and increased milk production in both rats and buffaloes.[32] One human study claimed that it was ineffective for increasing milk production and had little effect on prolactin. However, the researchers used only a very small dose, did not measure prolactin reliably, and also combined shatavari with other herbs, casting considerable doubt on their conclusions.[33] Shatavari has been favorably compared to metoclopramide for gastric problems and appears to cause a similar increase in prolactin, which could explain how it might help to increase milk.[34] It's unknown if it overlaps or adds to the way other medications and herbs increase prolactin. Shatavari is also reputed to block oxytocin receptors in the uterus, which may be why the Ayurvedic tradition considers it useful for preventing miscarriage or premature labor.[35] *Note: because animal research has shown some problems with fetal development, we don't recommend its use during pregnancy at this time.* While it may seem that this could interfere with milk ejection, such complaints have not been found. In an informal survey conducted on our website, three-quarters of mothers with a variety of situations reported an increase in milk production, and some even weaned from domperidone to shatavari, maintaining most of their milk supply. Few side effects were reported, although several mentioned breast tenderness, breast enlargement, and increases in vaginal fluid and sex drive.

Vervain (*Verbena Officinalis*). Another lactogenic herb with diuretic properties, European vervain may also stimulate uterine contractions, so it isn't used during pregnancy. Vervain is not one of the more commonly used galactogogues but does have a historical reputation for increasing milk production by Europeans and Native Americans.

Using Herbs to Increase Milk Supply During Pregnancy

If you want to continue breastfeeding during a new pregnancy, especially if your current nursling is very young, a galactogogue may help maintain some of your milk production. However, you're working against nature; your body's first priority is to prepare for the new baby. A decrease in volume and return to colostrum-type milk is normal.

Not all herbal galactogogues are appropriate for pregnancy, especially those that are reputed to have oxytocic/uterine stimulating effects. Those generally considered safe for pregnancy include red raspberry, nettle, oat straw, dandelion leaf, alfalfa, fennel, and milk thistle.

Maybe you had milk production problems in the past and are now pregnant again and wondering if taking a galactogogue during pregnancy would increase your odds. This is not an easy question to answer because it hasn't been researched. Depending on the root problem, some galactogogues such as alfalfa might help build milk-making tissue when the milk glands did not seem to respond with normal growth during the previous pregnancy.

Commercial Herbal Products

There are several good commercial galactogogue products on the market in North America that can work well in a number of circumstances. Although they have not been reviewed by the FDA for effectiveness and are not regulated in the same way as drugs, herbs used as dietary supplements do fall under the FDA's "food

185

and spice" category. They must meet the same basic standards for sterilization and handling, and their packaging can't contain unproven health claims. See www.lowmilksupply.org for detailed information on specific products.

Nursing Tea Combinations. Historically, most herbs were brewed into teas, and remedies for increasing milk production were no exception. Galactogogue teas are preferred by many herbalists for the comforting ritual of their preparation. Many lactation consultants consider lactation teas to be milder in effect than tinctures or capsules, but that may depend on using the right amount and preparing it properly. Katherine Shealy, M.P.H., IBCLC, experimented and observed that some teas are more effective if taken *eight to nine cups a day* rather than the recommended two to three cups. She also developed a tasty flavored version brewed in an iced tea maker for her neonatal intensive care unit (NICU) mothers to sip on throughout the day, eliminating the work of making multiple individual cups of tea. Her recipe: Brew 6 bags of Traditional Medicinals Mother's Milk tea plus 4 bags of Celestial Seasonings Wild Berry Zinger tea to make 3 quarts (2.8 liters). Pour into two 2-quart (1.9-liter) water bottles and drink throughout the day.

Various commercial brands offer slightly different herb combinations. Steeping time is very important for the proper diffusion of the herbs into the tea; too short will make a less effective product. Covering the tea during steeping helps to prevent evaporation of the water soluble components into the air. While some products call for only five minutes of steeping time, a minimum of ten minutes may result in a more effective product.

Nursing Tinctures. There are several combination galactogogue tinctures on the market that can be very effective. A few companies offer them commercially, while there are also several small mom-and-pop businesses that offer their own combinations for sale. Some are tinctures of just one herb, and others are blends of herbs specifically combined for their lactogenic properties. Most are alcohol-based (the small amount ingested is not a problem), though some are available in glycerin form. Tinctures may be made from fresh or dried herbs, and this can affect the potency as well as the price. Remember that suggested dosages are not set in stone. You may need more or less, depending on your situation.

Commercial Galactogogue Capsules. While most combinations come in the form of tinctures, some companies have placed their blends into capsules to eliminate unpleasant tastes and make dosing easier. Vitanica's Lactation Blend and TTK's Lactare (from India) are made from dried herbs, while Motherlove Herbal's More Milk Plus contains concentrated glycerin-based tincture.

Customizing Your Own Blend

Creating your own combination is another alternative and provides the opportunity to tailor the herbs to your situation. Some mothers have created their own tinctures, and others have simply bought bulk herbs to make a custom tea or decoction blend. Although we often correctly assume that multiple herbs will add to a stronger overall effect or at least help each other, keep in mind that *there is also the possibility that they may cancel out some of each other's properties, negating the advantage.* You may want to try herbs one at a time and then try combining them to see if the effect is better or simply overlapping. Why use (or spend) more than you need?

After struggling and never making quite enough milk for her first baby, "Cindy" researched and created her own special blend of herbs. For pregnancy, she devised a bulk tea mix to enhance her mammary gland growth made from a generous handful each of red raspberry leaf and nettle, and slightly smaller amounts of alfalfa and red clover. She added a handful of this mix to 1 quart (946 milliliters) of almost boiling water and allowed it to steep overnight. Cindy drank one cup each day during the first trimester and worked up to a quart a day by the end of pregnancy. Once the baby was born, she added other herbs that would enhance milk supply to her mix: handfuls of hops flower, blessed thistle, and marshmallow root. When she made a batch, she added a heaping teaspoon (5 milliliters) each of fenugreek powder and goat's rue powder to the pot. She continued to drink a quart a day, usually iced to mask the bitterness of some of the herbs (sweeteners can be used, too). She credits her "lactation brew" for her full supply with her next baby. For Cindy and a few other mothers, this selection of herbs seemed to be helpful. It is important to remember, however, that *there is no one magic combination that is perfect for everyone.*

Herbal Galactogogue Resources

There are many companies that market herbal galactogogues, but those that we have found to have high-quality products include Motherlove Herbal Company (www.motherlove.com), Wise Woman Herbals (www.wisewomanherbals.com), Nature's Way (www.naturesway .com), Traditional Medicinals (www.traditionalmedicinals.com), Mountain Rose Herbs (www.mountainroseherbs.com), Pure Herbs Ltd (www.pureherbs.com), and Birth and Breastfeeding Resources (www.birthandbreastfeeding.com). Ayurceutics (www.ayurceutics .com) carries certified heavy metal–free shatavari and ashwagandha, and Organic Partners (www.organicpartners.com) carries certified heavy metal–free shatavari.

Milk Ejection Aids

The ability to remove milk is as important as being able to make it. Pharmaceutical remedies for milk ejection have been limited to synthetic oxytocin (Pitocin). Syntocinon®, a nasal spray preparation of oxytocin, is no longer commercially available, but a similar product can be prepared by a pharmacist with a doctor's prescription. The usual dosage is one spray (three drops) in each nostril two to three minutes before breastfeeding or pumping. The use of synthetic oxytocin to aid milk ejection is usually temporary and rarely required for longer than a week. Though past research appears to validate the usefulness of oxytocin nasal spray to increase milk flow and thus production, a more recent study involving women who were not all having problems did not find it helpful.[36] It seems likely that synthetic oxytocin probably works for women with genuine milk ejection problems.

There are several herbs with varying reputations for helping with milk ejection. When stress is a factor, chamomile, usually tea, is well known for its calming effects and is sometimes taken before nursing to help mother relax and release her milk. There are also a few galactogogue herbs that have additional reputations for helping with milk ejection, though it is difficult to tell if they help with the actual ejection or if they help ejection by increasing milk volume (the fuller the water balloon, the faster the water comes out!). These include anise, black cohosh, blackseed, chasteberry, dill, fennel, hops, and red raspberry leaf. Lactation consultant Margie Deutsch-Lash, IBCLC, prefers red raspberry leaf tincture, 1 milliliter held under the tongue for thirty seconds before swallowing, ten minutes before a feeding, but says that if a mother likes tea better, it is best taken twenty minutes before feeding as it is absorbed more slowly in the stomach.

Commercially, there are two products that are used to aid milk ejection. The first is a flower essence tincture known as Rescue Remedy, recommended by many lactation consultants for its calming effect that seems to facilitate the milk ejection reflex. Several different manufacturers produce it, typically combining cherry plum, impatiens, rock rose, and star of Bethlehem. A few drops placed under the tongue for absorption right before breastfeeding is the usual dose. The second tincture product, Let-Down Formula, was created by Mechell Turner for Birth and Breastfeeding Resources especially to aid milk ejection. It includes schizandra berries, black cohosh, and motherwort.

Homeopathic Galactogogues

Homeopathy is a healing philosophy that is counterintuitive to Western medicine. The prescription of homeopathic remedies/medicines is based on the ancient Law of Similars, or "like treats like," rather than the Western approach of treating a problem with something designed to counteract it. Homeopathy interprets physical and emotional signs and symptoms as the means by which the body is trying to restore order when it is out of balance and so facilitates the choice of a medicine capable of actually causing that same particular set of signs and symptoms as a way to assist the body in its attempts to heal.

Some homeopathic remedies can be used generally for particular problems, but ideally they are chosen by an experienced practitioner after a detailed screening of your history and situation. The homeopathic approach is complex and not easily reduced to a list or table of remedies as there are dozens of possible remedies depending on what the practitioner determines the root problems to be.

Because homeopathy doesn't easily fit into the Western paradigm of medicine, it is difficult to list homeopathic galactogogues in an absolute sense. There are some that are appropriate for general application to low milk production, while the vast majority require specific tailoring to a mother's unique situation. Remedies/medicines usually come in X (1:10), C (1:100), or LM (1:50,000) potencies and may be liquid or pills. For use without the advice of a practitioner, 6C or 12C dilutions are usually most appropriate.

In order to save on medicine and effect the smoothest possible healing response, homeopath Patricia Hatherly, B.H.Sc.(Hom), IBCLC, suggests placing either three pills or three drops of the remedy into a small bottle (300 to 500 milliliters) of spring water and taking a teaspoon (5 milliliters) three times a day, shaking the bottle in between.

Table 3 in the appendix lists several of the many homeopathic remedies that may be used for low milk production in various situations. For best results, it is wise to consult an experienced practitioner as they are skilled at choosing the most appropriate prescription for your unique situation.

When Do I Stop Taking a Galactogogue?

The appropriate time to stop taking galacogogues depends on your circumstances. In most cases of uncomplicated low milk supply, you can start weaning down as soon as you've reached full production and baby is able to sustain it. Reduce your galactogogues gradually; otherwise, you'll probably experience a drop in milk production. If your body seems to be struggling, such as with an iron deficiency, a hormonal problem, or a lack of sufficient breast tissue, the galactogogue may be required for weeks or months or possibly even the entire time you're breastfeeding. Sometimes the body seems to "kick in" after a time of additional support, while other times the breast needs the support permanently. When the use becomes long-term, some find that they are able to cut back some, if not completely, around six months or so when their baby starts to eat solids. You can always try slowly reducing your dosage and/or frequency, no more than 25 percent every week, and if you begin to experience a drop in milk production, just start back up again.

CHAPTER 13

Making More Milk When You Return to Work or School

Throughout time, mothers have worked, continued their education, and pursued volunteer activities while successfully breastfeeding their children. Women today not only have the benefit of their wisdom, but they also have new resources and technology to increase their success. Whether you are starting out with milk production that is already low or have low milk production challenges as a result of returning to work or school, this chapter will help you find strategies to make the most milk possible for your baby. To simplify, we'll call all mothers separated regularly from their babies "working mothers," but we understand that your "work" is not always in a traditional job.

Maximizing Your Milk Production

Your best chance for continuing to breastfeed successfully is to invest the time to establish maximum milk production before you go back. The higher you can calibrate your initial milk production, the more resilient it will be if you have difficulties later on.

As mentioned in Chapter 5, it may help to pump several times a day in addition to breastfeeding for at least the first two to three weeks to deliberately overstimulate your production and create a cushion for the inevitable bumps down the road. For a maternity leave of six weeks or less, continue to pump as many times a day as you can. For a leave of two months or longer, hold off pumping until a week or so before you return, or you can pump once a day whenever milk production is at its highest point. Any milk pumped now can be stockpiled in your freezer as insurance for later.

You may not get a lot in the beginning. Don't think that means you'll have problems making enough milk when returning to work. Your baby has simply taken all the available milk, and there's not much left to pump. The point of using the pump is to tell your breasts to make more than they're currently making. When you're pumping in lieu of breastfeeding, there will be plenty of milk.

As you work to maximize your milk production, keep your time with baby in the forefront, because those first few weeks fly by quickly. Yes, you need to plan for the day you have to go back to work or school, but don't spend so much time preparing and stressing about it that you miss out on this precious chance to bond with your baby. You'll produce more milk and make the transition back to work more easily if you put baby first and fit preparations in as you go.

Make Your Plan

Before you return, you'll need a plan for how to manage breast-feeding while you are away from your baby. Keep it flexible so you can adapt to the unexpected. There is no single right approach because situations and childcare options vary. The main factors that affect your plan are how long you'll be away from baby, how close your caregiver is, and what your baby will be fed during the workday.

Some moms choose not to pump at all while they are away from baby, breastfeeding only at night and on weekends and having the sitter give formula instead. This creates a challenge for keeping milk production up, especially if the time away is long, but a number of mothers have done it successfully. The key is making sure to breastfeed as much as possible when you and baby are together. If you want your baby to have only your milk, or at least as much of it as possible, you'll need to express milk for when you aren't together. Just like the first few weeks after baby was born, returning to work or school may be a little bit awkward as you find your way and settle into a routine. The following recommendations will help minimize the impact on your milk production.

Get a Good Pump

While some mothers are very skilled at hand expressing, most find it more efficient and time-effective to use a high-quality pump with a dual kit when away from baby. If you start with a good supply, a high-end consumer pump is usually sufficient; but if you struggle with milk production, a hospital-grade pump is a wiser choice. Shop until you find one that you really like; it's worth the investment. For helpful information on choosing a pump, see Chapter 11.

Plan Your Schedule

To know how many times you'll need to pump each day, pay attention to how many times baby normally feeds during the time period you'll be away from him. Aim for fitting in that many pumping sessions, adding extra opportunities for feeding and pumping into your schedule to help keep your supply up.

Here's an example for an eight-hour day: Before it's time to get up, wake baby for a leisurely feeding in bed while you rest for a few more minutes. With his tummy full, baby should be content while you get ready for the day. Give him a "top off" feeding right before you leave home or at the sitter's. If you have time, pump as soon as you get to work or school even though you may have nursed just a short while before. Then pump during your morning, lunch, and afternoon breaks. Ask your caregiver not to feed baby close to the time you're due to arrive so that he'll be ready to eat when you pick him up or right when you get home. Should you be late, baby can be given just an ounce or so to keep him happy so he's still hungry when you get there. Nurse baby once or twice in the evening, right before he goes to sleep, and at least once during the night.

By now you've fit more than eight sessions of pumping or nursing into your day! Even though you've been away from baby for eight to ten hours, you're still nursing or pumping as many times as mothers who are with their babies full-time. That's going to go a long way toward keeping your milk production high. Of course, there will be days when fitting in all those nursing and pumping sessions just can't happen. Doing your best to breastfeed and pump as often as you can will keep your milk production as high as possible.

When you're with baby, make breastfeeding a high priority. Many mothers set a rule that baby gets bottles only when they are at work, and all the rest of the time they commit to breastfeeding. Resist the temptation to let someone else feed a bottle of pumped milk just because it's already prepared and handy and you have something else you need to do. Giving a bottle of milk instead of nursing decreases your supply by that amount, so bottles should be given only when you aren't with him. Plus, too many bottles can lead to breast refusal if baby spends more time with the bottle than the breast. On evenings and weekends, keep baby with you wherever you go so you can nurse when he wants to, even at the movies or out to dinner.

Creative Schedules

Don't overlook creative scheduling possibilities. Can you minimize the time you and baby are separated? How about working or going to school part-time at first? Or taking online classes or working from home? Can baby come with you for some or all of the time, at least in the early weeks or months? Can baby be brought to you, or can you go to baby, for at least one nursing each day? Could you take part or all of Wednesday off so that you have to rely on pumping to maintain your milk supply for only two days at a time? Would fewer longer days or more shorter days work better in your situation? Think creatively and don't hesitate to express your needs to those who can help, especially your employer or professors.

How Milk Production Can Decrease

It's so common to hear about working mothers having problems with their milk supplies that it seems inevitable. Milk production may start off very well at the beginning of the week but lag by the end. A pumping routine that works well on Monday may not produce the same amount of milk on Thursday or Friday. Other times, mothers find that milk production seems to decrease around two to three months. These experiences aren't inevitable, but there are many reasons they can happen.

Pumping Frequency

The most likely suspect when a working mother's milk supply drops is a decrease in pumping. If your job or class schedule keeps you running most of the day, it can be difficult to fit in enough pumping sessions. You may start off expressing three or four times each day but eventually find that you're pumping only a couple of times at most on busy days, and there seem to be more busy days than not. One solution may be to use a hands-free kit (see Chapter 11) so you can multitask while pumping. Another idea is to schedule pumping time on your day planner, PDA, or shared calendar. If you don't have enough time for a full pumping session, *it's better to pump for even a few minutes than not at all.* Anything is better than nothing.

What if your pumping schedule hasn't changed but baby starts sleeping longer at night so he's nursing less when you're with him? It might seem great at first because you're getting more rest. But baby has to make up those feedings in some way, and it's probably going to be during the day at the sitter's. To keep up with his need for more milk then, you'll need to either add in another one or two pumping sessions, wake baby for an additional feed right before you go to bed, or reconsider the value of uninterrupted sleep. If baby can be encouraged to nurse at least once during the night, you can minimize the effort of night feeding by having him sleep with you or near you for the next few months.

One last possibility when frequency is an issue is how you determine when it's time to pump. Do you wait until your breasts feel full? That can lead to longer and longer pumping intervals because milk is made most slowly when the breast is full.

Travel

Everything can be going along wonderfully until you're called away on a trip out of town, wreaking havoc with your pumping schedule, let alone finding ways to store the milk you pump while you're away. You may need to think creatively to work around any travel-related obstacles.

Diana Cassar-Uhl, an instrumentalist in the U.S. Military Academy Band at West Point, La Leche League Leader, and mother of three exclusively breastfed children, has dealt with her extensive travel schedule by having an au pair accompany her and the baby on trips. Of course, this can be expensive and isn't always possible, but it's one option to consider. A family member such as a grandma can also be a boon in such situations.

If you are worried about hauling around your electric pump or power sources for it, bring a manual pump; they can be used almost anywhere. Some mothers find a way to store the milk and bring it home. On long trips, determined mothers have even shipped milk home. But another option is to "pump and dump." It seems a shame to waste it, but it keeps your supply up. Whichever you choose, just keep the milk flowing.

Caregiver Feeding Methods

You may think there's a problem with your milk supply because your caregiver is telling you that your baby needs more milk during the day than you're sending in. But if the amount you're making hasn't changed, the problem is more likely to do with how your sitter is feeding your baby.

Is she offering a bottle as a first resort when baby fusses? Most babies will take a bottle even when the problem isn't hunger. What they really need is the cuddling that comes with the feeding. Encourage your sitter to try other ways to soothe baby than just reaching for a bottle. Is baby taking more and more milk? Babies will usually take more if it's offered even if they don't really need more. Your sitter may not know that breastfed babies don't need ever-increasing amounts of milk like formula-fed babies do because their metabolic needs are different. Have you upgraded to a nipple size larger than "newborn" or "slow flow"? Has the sitter cut the opening to make it flow faster? Breastfed babies should stay at the slowest flow nipple so the flow is similar to the breast, to avoid flow preference (see Chapter 4). How is baby gaining? If he's gaining more weight than normal, it is a clear sign he's being given too much to eat.

Is the feeding being ended when baby seems satisfied, or is he being encouraged to finish the bottle so none is wasted? Find out if any milk is being thrown away at the end (and if so, how much), and let her know that unlike formula, your milk lasts longer and may be usable for a couple of hours. It also may help to send the milk in smaller increments so that it is used only as needed.

Is baby being fed in a mostly upright position? If not, the milk can flow so quickly that baby may still root for more, not realizing he's already full. Demonstrate how to pace the feeding by periodically leaning baby forward for a break; this will help both your caregiver and baby learn to regulate the feeding naturally (see Chapter 4). Reassure her that it won't prolong the feeding, and it may reduce the need for burping. A helpful article that you can print out and share with your caregiver can be found at www .kellymom.com/bf/pumping/bottle-feeding.html.

Growth Spurts

Even when the sitter feeds baby in all the right ways, there will be days when baby goes through all the milk you pumped the day before by noon and nurses nonstop when you get home. He's probably going through a growth spurt and will want more milk than usual until it passes. During this time, you may need to add an extra pumping or two to keep up. If that isn't possible, it's a good time to dip into your frozen stockpile if you have one. Fortunately, it should last for only two to three days, and then he'll be back to the normal amount.

It Isn't Always About Work

What if you're pumping often enough with a great pump and your caregiver isn't overfeeding but there's still not enough milk? First, rule out any other management-related, baby-sided, or structural problems described in Chapters 6 through 8. Is it possible that you're pregnant? Have you taken any decongestants or new medications or eaten a lot of mint candy, tabouleh, or sage? Have you started taking hormonal birth control? Has baby started sleeping through the night? If nothing fits, the problem may be hormonal. Were you able to maximize your milk production capability by removing as much milk as possible in the first few weeks? If not, you may not have enough receptors, which may be affecting your milk production now. Look in Chapter 9 for possible causes, particularly thyroid problems, and if necessary, make an appointment with your doctor to discuss your concerns.

Pump Effectiveness

The second most likely suspect when a working mother's milk production decreases is her pump. How good is the one you're using? Most working mothers need a high-end pump to remove their milk effectively. Make sure your flanges fit well and all the connections are correct. Try adjusting the cycling speed either up or down to better match the way your baby nurses. If you're using a consumer-grade pump, how old is it? As explained in Chapter 11, they're not designed to work at top efficiency for much longer than a year and can deteriorate so slowly that you may not notice. If you used it with your last baby or you borrowed it from someone else, try renting a pump for a week to see if you get more milk. If so, maybe you need to invest in a new pump. It may also help to read back through Chapter 11 for tips to increase your pumping output.

Increasing Your Supply While Working

The faster you take action to correct a decrease in milk production, the easier it will be to bring it back up. Don't hesitate, hoping that it will get better on its own. Addressing the cause now will help things get back to normal sooner. If the problem is due to a faulty pump or scheduling problems, the following ideas may help.

Increase Frequency

One of the most effective ways to compensate for a decrease in pumping output is to spend your weekend "power nursing" your baby. Encourage him to nurse often to rebuild your supply for the new week. If baby doesn't want to nurse more often or other things interfere, "power pumping" as described in Chapter 11 can accomplish the same result.

Breast Compressions

Try using breast compressions to increase the amount of milk that you can remove while pumping. As described in Chapter 5, breast compressions are a way to add pressure inside the breast so the milk flows more forcibly through the ducts, almost like creating another milk ejection.

Reverse Cycling

Seeking to avoid the pressure of pumping enough milk for day-time feedings while working the demanding schedule of a resident, Dr. Marilyn Grams developed a unique strategy that she calls "reverse cycling": deliberately feed more at night than during the day. She discovered that when she encouraged lots of night-time nursings, her baby needed less pumped milk during the day. She also found that she was able to maintain a strong supply under challenging work circumstances. The quality of her rest didn't suffer because she learned to nurse comfortably while lying down and to sleep through the feedings. It's a counterintuitive strategy that has worked well for many working mothers and is worth trying. Babies have also been known to initiate this themselves, taking little at the sitter's and waiting until mom returns, after which they start feeding in earnest.

If you're worried about sleep, go to bed an hour or two earlier than usual (after feeding) and let your partner care for baby so you can sleep alone for a while. On weekend mornings, have your partner get up with baby (after feeding) so you can go back to sleep. Nap with baby whenever possible.

Milk Ejection Remedies

After several weeks or months nursing your baby before you returned to work, your milk ejection was conditioned to happen when he breastfed. It can take some adjustment to make it happen when you turn the pump on.

Since the sense of smell has an amazing power to trigger a physical reaction, try holding your baby's unwashed blanket or clothing next to your face as you pump. An iPod recording of his gurgling, coos, or gentle cries, or even a picture of him may elicit the same response. If you have a special song that you sing to your baby, try humming it to yourself as you pump. On the other hand, some mothers find that reminders of their baby actually keep the milk ejection from happening because they miss him so much.

Samantha Leeson, a doula in Ontario, had never felt milk ejection with her first son, Fergus, or her new baby, Quinn, so when she returned to work, she found it difficult to know what to do to let down to the pump. One night, she tried nursing Quinn on one side and pumping on the other at the same time. This gave her a guide for timing and helped her transition from Quinn to the pump. After doing this several times, she was able to have a milk ejection while pumping without needing Quinn to help.

If privacy is the issue, see if you can find either a more secluded place to pump (*not* the bathroom!) or a way to make your pumping place more private. Can you put up a sign to discourage visitors? Can you install a lock on the door? Can you hang curtains? Can you go to your car? There are also many other ideas for enhancing milk ejection in Chapter 10.

Consider Galactagogues

If you've done your best to maximize milk removal but are still falling short, galactogogues may help fill the gap. For a modest boost, one great idea is to brew and ice a pitcher of a nursing mother's tea in the morning and sip on it throughout the day. See Chapter 12 for more ideas.

Solids Take the Pressure Off

Once baby begins taking solids, they can be used as part of baby's supplement at the sitter's. This will begin to take the pressure off how much milk you need to provide each day. Of course, solids should be offered only in small amounts at first, so this transition will be very gradual. When given at home, be sure to breastfeed first so he fills up on your milk. However, when your sitter gives baby solids, they should be given *before* the bottle to reduce his need for milk while you are away.

Making More Milk in Special Situations: Exclusive Pumping, Premies, Multiples, Relactation, and Induced Lactation

Coping with low milk production is difficult even in the best of circumstances. At times, mothers are faced with additional challenges such as exclusive pumping, premies, multiples, relactation, or induced lactation for a surrogate-born or adopted baby who requires specialized strategies to increase milk production.

Exclusive Pumping

Long-term pumping and bottle-feeding happen for a variety of reasons. You may have had problems that made feeding at the breast difficult or impossible. Or you may want the best for your baby but don't want to breastfeed. Exclusive pumping challenges milk production because the infant has been taken out of the equation. Even when given human milk, babies fed by bottle tend to develop feeding patterns that are different from how they would have breastfed, so baby's eating pattern is not always the best guide for developing an appropriate pumping routine for your body. Nor does the same schedule work equally well for every exclusively pumping mother. Some mothers are able to sustain pumping large amounts of milk in just a few sessions a day, while others need to pump more often to maintain adequate production. It's wiser to pump more frequently in the early weeks and store any extra milk in the freezer than cut back too quickly to the fewest number of sessions necessary to obtain a certain amount of milk. Eventually, you may be able to get by with fewer pumping sessions, but for the first several weeks, shoot for pumping at least eight times per twenty-four hours. Rather than pumping at certain intervals, you're likely to get more milk by keeping the amount of time in between pumpings as short as possible so the breasts don't get overly full and slow down production.

After the first three or four weeks, you can experiment to determine how often and how long it is necessary to pump to have enough milk for your baby.[1] All breasts respond differently, so pay attention to how your breasts feel and not just the clock. When most of the available milk has been removed, they'll feel soft and light. After pumping a few times, you'll learn what this feels like. Sometimes it will take longer, sometimes shorter. And sometimes you'll pump past that point to provide extra stimulation. Pumping intuitively will keep your pumping routine efficient.

If you're having difficulty meeting baby's daily needs, first make sure he isn't being overfed. If not, power pumping or increasing the number of pumping sessions per day may help increase your supply. The suggestions for effective pumping in Chapter 11 as well as many of the strategies suggested for working mothers in Chapter 13 may help. Galactogogues are most effective when there is frequent milk removal to go with them.

Exclusive pumping for an extended time period requires dedication, and sometimes it can be hard to stay motivated. Connecting to other mothers who are exclusively pumping through an online e-mail support group such as PumpMoms (www.pump ingmoms.org) may make all the difference. The Ameda web-site also offers helpful and supportive information (www.ameda .com/breastpumping/moms).

Premature Babies

When a baby is born prematurely, lactation rarely begins normally because of the events surrounding the early birth. A small but otherwise healthy baby may be able to breastfeed soon, but chances are good that he may not be strong enough to get all his nourishment from the breast right away. Quite often, premature babies are not ready to breastfeed at all after birth; the earlier they come, the more likely this is true. So you will need to start pumping as soon and as frequently as possible to establish good milk production.

One question is whether the breast is "fully operational" for mothers who deliver prematurely. Because the basic glandular structures are complete by the first half of pregnancy, it has been assumed that full milk production is possible. However, this may not be true for all mothers, especially when delivering between twenty-two and thirty-four weeks of gestation.[2] Milk-making cells enlarge during the second half of pregnancy, and the impact of shortening this growth time was unknown before now. But new research is showing that milk volume in the beginning is directly related to gestational age at birth and rises as gestational age increases.[3]

Another new insight is a previously unnoticed relationship between the use of corticosteroids such as betamethasone and a delay in milk production after birth. These drugs are often given when premature delivery threatens because they can improve the baby's ability to cope and survive. The amount of time between the treatment and the birth seems to make a difference; from zero to two days the effect was small, but from three to nine days it was much greater.[4]

Finally, there is the question of why baby was born early, because preexisting medical or infertility conditions that can result in premature births might also subtly affect the developing breast. If your baby was small for gestational age (SGA), intrauterine growth restricted (IUGR), or a problem with the placenta was suspected, be sure to read about placental problems in Chapter 9 and remember that breast tissue can still be built up after birth.

You may not have much control over the physical factors, but there are other things under your control that can make a big difference because the rule of demand and supply is still in effect. In the first week, mothers who give birth prematurely often start off producing the same amount of milk as mothers who give birth at term but may end up with much less milk than full-term mothers after six weeks. The difference lies in *how often* premie mothers pump compared to how often the other mothers breastfeed.[5] *To be most successful, it's best to pump frequently (eight or more times per day) from the beginning and ignore the temptation to try and get by with less.* The tiny premie who at first needs only a few ounces of milk per day will eventually grow and develop a bigger appetite, and his mother needs to establish a milk supply for his future as a larger baby.

A good pumping goal is at least 16 ounces (500 milliliters) per day, but preferably 25 to 33 ounces (750 to 1,000 milliliters) by two weeks postpartum to attain a full supply.[6] If you don't reach this range, just keep working steadily and perhaps consider a galactogogue. When milk production seems to fluctuate significantly at times, take a look at what else is going on in your life. It's not uncommon for the amount of milk you pump to drop temporarily if you receive distressing news about your baby. This usually rebounds when baby improves and you're feeling better again. Mothers of very ill babies are under a tremendous amount of pressure, and it's understandable that occasionally this may affect your milk ejection.

The day you are able to put your precious baby to your breast for the first time will be a moment for the scrapbook! You may need to continue pumping for top-off feedings or just as insurance, since premie babies often don't do the best job of keeping milk production going until they get bigger. Once he becomes a proficient feeder, you'll need to pump or use galactagogues only if you haven't reached a full supply. Otherwise, you can gradually wean away from pumping.

Multiples

Supporting a single baby can seem challenging enough, but when you have twins or more, milk supply worries can double or triple! Fortunately, most mothers who give birth to multiples are able to produce enough milk for twins and even triplets or more.[7] Animal studies show that the more total placental weight, the more mammary gland development occurs during the pregnancy.[8] This appears to be equally true for human mothers. So the fact that you had two or more babies is itself a bonus—your starting milk factory is likely to be larger than if you had only one baby.[9]

Still, it's common for mothers of multiples to have concerns about their milk production. If you've been nursing your babies exclusively, it's important to carefully evaluate their milk intake to know for sure if there's a problem. Each baby's weight gain and diaper output should be considered independently. If one is doing well but another is not, it may be that the baby who is not getting enough milk is not being brought to the breast often enough or is not allowed to nurse long enough, perhaps because he is a more leisurely breastfeeder than his sibling. It's also possible that one baby may not be removing milk from the breast efficiently due to immature, disorganized suckling patterns; he may need supplementation until he matures. Or he may have a tongue restriction problem that requires evaluation and treatment. In the meantime, you may want to alternate the breast from which each baby is fed in order to ensure that both breasts receive equal amounts of stimulation, and pump for the baby who isn't able to remove sufficient milk yet. If the suck of one or more of your babies isn't yet effective, which commonly happens because multiples are often born early and with varying degrees of maturity, Chapter 7 will help you explore possible causes, but a visit with a lactation consultant is often helpful.

When multiples are born prematurely and you must pump until the babies are able to nurse, there is a greater risk of having problems with low milk production. The pumping routine normally used to establish a milk supply for one baby must now create milk for two babies. If this doesn't happen, milk production may not calibrate high enough. If one or both babies are at home from the hospital, use the strategies in Chapter 4 for supplementing in a way that is supportive of breastfeeding as you work to increase your milk production.

Begin pumping as soon after birth as possible, preferably within the first hour, with a goal of eight or more fifteen-minute double-pumping sessions per day. Trying to fit in that many pumping sessions when you are also visiting your babies in the hospital each day can be difficult, so don't worry about spacing pumping sessions evenly; it's fine to cluster some of them closer together, just as your babies are likely to cluster some of the feedings together when they begin nursing. Keep in mind that when you first start pumping more frequently, you are likely to see less milk in each pumping session, but the total amount will be the same, and higher later on. See Chapter 11 for tips to enhance your milk output.

Once both babies are able to breastfeed, you may be able to discontinue pumping, depending on how effectively each breastfeeds. If you aren't sure, a little extra "insurance pumping" will guarantee that the breasts are drained well and adequately stimulated. But, if the babies aren't removing milk effectively overall, it's better for both your sanity and milk production to spend more time on pumping and less on breastfeeding until they can nurse better.

Simultaneous nursing can be a real time-saver, with the added advantage that the babies can help each other in stimulating milk ejections. It doesn't work well for everyone, but it's worth giving a try. There's no rush; wait until at least one baby is able to latch and nurse effectively before you attempt both babies together. It may be easier to first latch the baby that has more difficulty.

If milk production is a struggle even though you've been doing "everything right," one additional thing to consider is whether the babies were conceived with or without fertility assistance. If there was a hormonal problem that affected your ability to conceive, it may now be affecting your milk production. (Addressing the specific hormonal problem, when possible, may improve lactation; see Chapter 9.) For more information about nursing multiples, read Karen Gromada's excellent book, *Mothering Multiples*, and visit her website, www.karengromada.com.

Relactation

Relactation is the process of rebuilding a milk supply weeks or months after baby stopped breastfeeding, which can happen for many reasons. Sometimes milk production appeared to be so low that it originally didn't seem worth the bother to continue breastfeeding. In other cases, doctors have told mothers they have to wean in order to take certain medications or undergo diagnostic tests, or just because breastfeeding has been a struggle and they don't know how to help. Long separations from baby or breast rejection can also lead to unintended weaning. Though it seemed like the right decision at the time, some women later regret their decision to wean and decide to reclaim their breastfeeding relationship. Or it simply may be that baby isn't tolerating formula and needs mother's milk.

In general, it may take about the same amount of time to resume exclusive breastfeeding as has elapsed since baby weaned, provided you once had a full supply. This means that if your baby was weaned a month ago, it may take up to a month to reestablish full milk production.

It can be reassuring to keep in mind that babies are born to breastfeed, and there are many ways to gently entice a baby back to the breast. Younger babies are usually more willing to return to nursing, but older babies have been known to take to it easily as well. For some, it may be necessary to get milk production back up before they'll agree to nurse. At-breast supplementers can help because they provide immediate satisfaction for baby's sucking effort. Or you also may find it helpful to give baby some milk by an alternate method before offering the breast (see Chapter

4). If he still won't latch, don't hesitate to enlist the help of an experienced lactation consultant, who may provide some helpful tips customized for your situation. Once baby is latching easily, avoid giving him a pacifier and encourage him to nurse at every opportunity.

The rate of milk production will increase more quickly if you're still in the early postpartum period than it will if you have an older baby. The less involution that has occurred, the better your chances for full relactation; however, the speed at which this happens varies and cannot be easily predicted.[10] If you had a full milk supply before baby stopped breastfeeding, you're more likely to recover it than if you had reached only a half supply before stopping. When weaning happens prior to six weeks postpartum, the breasts may not have had a chance to fully develop the milk-making tissue and hormone receptors.

"Relactation boot camp" is promoted on some Internet websites, but it involves nothing more than very frequent nursing, similar to a "babymoon" or "nursing vacation," and isn't likely to provide baby with enough milk in the short term when your milk production is low or nonexistent. The technique advises eating a very healthy diet and consuming large quantities of fluid even though increased nutrition, calories, and hydration have not been shown to have a significant effect on the amount of milk produced unless the mother is extremely malnourished or dehydrated, as discussed in Chapter 6. Frequent nursing and a positive "can do" attitude can certainly help, but supplementation combined with effective methods to increase milk production beyond baby's sucking, such as pumping with a hospital-grade pump and using galactagogues, are usually necessary.

Induced Lactation

Induced lactation is the process of creating a milk supply for a child you have not birthed. With a long historical tradition in native societies, it is becoming more common as women learn that it is possible.[11] For both adoptive mothers and mothers of surrogate babies, breastfeeding is about more than the milk—it's a way to connect at a deeper level with your new baby and contribute to his growth beyond the pregnancy. Although it will require time, motivation, perseverance, tenacity, and patience, breastfeeding your baby can be tremendously rewarding.

As with relactation, the younger the baby, the more likely he is to latch onto the breast easily. A baby older than three months is liable to have more difficulty learning what to do than a newborn. All babies nurse more willingly when there is more milk, so it helps to do all you can to maximize your production. Achieving a full supply may be possible provided there aren't underlying problems such as hormonal dysfunctions or underdeveloped breast tissue. If you struggled with infertility in particular, there may be a hormonal problem that could limit your milk-making capability. However, most mothers can make at least some milk, and the total amount of milk need not interfere with a satisfying breastfeeding relationship. While you won't produce true colostrum, the milk you make will be the same quality as a birth mother's mature milk.[12]

If you're currently nursing but want to breastfeed a new baby you did not birth, you may not be able to increase milk production enough to meet the new baby's needs fully because you are in the autumn season of lactation now. But it's always worth trying because your new baby will benefit from whatever extra you can make.

Methods of Inducing Milk Production

In traditional cultures, women have successfully stimulated milk production just by putting the baby to the breast very frequently. Our Western approach relies more often on breast pump technology, but pumping is an imperfect way to induce milk production because it is cold, mechanical, and vacuum-centered only. Plus, it takes time to become comfortable and proficient at pumping. Even birth mothers with excellent milk production aren't always able to pump effectively, especially in the beginning. A nursing baby adds a positive emotional element; not only does suckling stimulate milk ejection, but the psychological effect of baby's smell, sight, and sounds triggers additional oxytocin releases that a pump cannot. If possible, combining pumping with nursing baby using an at-breast supplementer can provide the best of both worlds. Adding galactogogue medications and/or herbs can result in significantly higher milk production.

Basic Pumping Protocol for Induced Lactation

1. Two to four weeks (or more) prior to the baby's arrival, begin manual massage of nipples and breasts for ten minutes eight to ten times per day for two weeks.

2. After two weeks, begin double pumping with a hospital-grade pump for ten to fifteen minutes eight to ten times per day. If you find pumping without a flow of milk to be uncomfortable, try putting a bit of breastfeeding-grade lanolin on your nipples or lubricate the funnel with a bit of vegetable or olive oil before pumping.

3. When baby arrives, use an at-breast supplementer to provide feedings at the breast (see Chapter 4). Pump after feedings or several times per day, as time permits (see "Power Pumping" in Chapter 11). Keep a close watch on baby's weight gain to ensure that he is getting enough nutrition.

4. As your breasts begin to feel full, heavy, and slightly tender, see if baby will nurse at the breast without supplementation for the first few minutes of the feeding if he is willing. Continue to watch diapers or track weight gain.

5. As long as hunger cues aren't frantic and weight gain is sufficient, gradually decrease either the amount of milk in the supplementer or the length of time the milk is allowed to flow from the supplementer during the feeding. Eventually, you may reach a point where you can no longer decrease the amount of supplement you offer without leaving baby hungry. That is the amount that will be needed for now, and maybe for the long term.

In the beginning, you have only your standby skeletal crew of lactocytes to start up milk production. Be patient. Induced lactation really is more like building a milk factory by hand from bricks and mortar instead of having the construction company, pregnancy, do it with all their specialized parts and equipment. Not as fancy and takes longer, but sooner or later new workers and assembly lines will slowly start to kick in, and your production will pick up.

Hormonal Simulation

Hormonal protocols for inducing lactation attempt to artificially simulate a pregnancy in order to build a milk factory. The amount of hormones used is less than what is normally produced during pregnancy. A birth control pill containing estrogen and progesterone is taken for a specific amount of time in order to stimulate the growth of more milk-making breast tissue. Then a prolactin-stimulating medication is introduced. Finally, pumping is begun to remove milk and further stimulate milk production.

In most cases, hormonal protocols result in more milk production than simple pumping. The more time you spend in the pregnancy-mimicking phase, the more milk-making tissue will be created. Starting at least four months before baby is expected to arrive produces the best results. You can initiate a protocol even after your baby arrives, but the shorter the lead time, the less you should expect to produce.

Milk does not come in until the pumping phase and first appears as clear drops that eventually become more opaque and white in color. As the milk volume increases, you may begin to see small sprays that eventually become streams of milk. The amount of time it takes to reach the streaming phase varies from mother to mother and depends on the type of protocol that she follows. It may take days, weeks, or months for milk production to begin. You'll know your body is gearing up to make milk when your breasts increase at least one bra cup size and feel full, heavy, and slightly tender. If you don't experience at least some tenderness within fifteen days, it may be necessary to increase your progesterone intake.

Because hormonal protocols entail the use of prescription drugs, it is essential to consult a physician. Present the entire protocol and explain that the birth control pill is not being used as a contraceptive but rather to develop lactation tissue. The medication can be started at any point in the menstrual cycle because the purpose is to simulate a pregnancy rather than prevent one.

Mothers who have blood clotting problems (a history of thrombosis), heart conditions, or severe blood pressure problems (hypertension) *should not* use hormonal protocols. Nor should mothers who wish to tandem nurse, because the existing milk supply will be reduced initially.

The Newman-Goldfarb protocols were developed by Lenore Goldfarb, B.Comm., B.Sc., IBCLC, in consultation with Dr. Jack Newman, as a result of her personal experience and subsequent work with other mothers, and are still evolving. They represent a new strategy that has not been formally tested in clinical trials but has been described theoretically by Dr. Peter Hartmann and his research group in Australia.[13] Many mothers have found the protocols to be effective. Similar but more limited protocols using medications to stimulate lactation hormones have been tested and found to be effective as well.[14]

There are several versions of the Newman-Goldfarb protocol to accommodate the varying amounts of time available before baby arrives and the mother's hormonal situation. Mothers who prepare for six months or more by following the "regular protocol" are more likely to induce a full milk supply, while mothers who do so for fewer than six months and follow the "accelerated protocol" are often able to induce a 50 percent supply. Mothers who follow the "menopause protocol" may produce a 25 percent or less milk supply.[15] Since these protocols are still evolving, visit the Ask Lenore website, www.asklenore.info/breastfeeding/abindex .html#protocols, for specific details and more information.

For more information about induced lactation, visit www .fourfriends.com/abrw, The Adoptive Breastfeeding Resource Website, and www.breast-feeding.adoption.com, Adoption.com's helpful section on breastfeeding.

Surviving the Present and Planning for the Future

"The Real Reason I Breastfeed" by Gina, mother of five

Because I have insufficient mammary tissue and have struggled with low milk production with all five of my babies, I have been asked many times, "Why do you bother? Why do you keep trying to breastfeed with all the problems you have?" I usually answer in several ways, such as, "It's better for my baby to have some breast milk than none" or "For bonding and closeness and visual and oral development." My favorite answer is, "Because breastfeeding is so much more than milk," but that answer is rarely understood. Well, the other day my little guy showed me how real that answer is. He had just finished nursing on one side and I straddled him on my lap while I situated the SNS. When I lifted my shirt, his eyes lit up, he smiled, and one hand went on each breast. He looked back and forth like a kid in a candy shop, trying to decide which one he wanted. His eyes were wide with excitement and he was full of giggles; it was so very cute! After several times of looking back and forth, he just plopped his head down and nestled between my breasts. He had one arm around each as if he was hugging them. This tender and sweet moment was the ultimate reward for a battle long fought, and the perfect illustration that "breastfeeding is so much more than milk." So why do I persevere despite the problems? The answer is easy . . . because it brings my baby joy and because my breasts offer more than milk. We aren't measured by the ounces in bottles but rather by the grit and determination behind those ounces. By that measure, none of us fail!

CHAPTER 15

Coping with Low Milk Supply

Most newly pregnant mothers today are aware of the importance of breastfeeding, often taking the ability to breastfeed for granted. But when that precious baby is born, the depth of emotions can be profound if you don't have enough milk or baby can't breastfeed well.

You have a choice about how you remember your breastfeeding experience by framing it in terms that are gratifying to you. This is not to say that you should dismiss or ignore negative feelings, but rather that it is important to find peace in your breastfeeding experience before too much time has passed so that negative feelings don't overflow into other areas of your life, especially your feelings about your baby's earliest days.

Making Peace with Your Milk Supply

No matter how you feel, you're not alone; other breastfeeding mothers have been down this road before you and felt the following emotions. Identifying, understanding, and processing them will give you peace.

Guilt or Regret

Some mothers feel guilt about decisions they made that affected the amount of milk they could produce, such as cosmetic breast surgery or using a poor-quality pump. Others feel as though they "starved" their baby before realizing he wasn't getting enough milk. Sometimes guilt is imposed on you by a doctor or family member who blames you for one thing or another. It's important to distinguish guilt from regret. Guilt assumes that you deliberately decided to do something knowing what the outcome would be. Regret happens after we learn something that we did not know at the time of the decision. Almost certainly, you made the best decisions with the information available to you at what was probably a very confusing time. *You did not know then what you know now or you might have made a different decision.* It's natural and healthy to feel regret because it helps us make better decisions in the future. But there is no need to entertain guilt when you didn't know what the outcome of your decision would be.

Anger and Resentment

Let's be honest—it isn't fair that some mothers have to work so much harder than others to breastfeed their babies. Anger and resentment are understandable feelings when breastfeeding doesn't happen the way you originally envisioned. When the problem is on your side, you may feel that your body let you down. Maybe a physician or family member was unsupportive or gave you inaccurate information that contributed to your difficulties. You may even feel anger toward your baby if he played a role in the problem, then feel guilty because you know that your baby doesn't understand and is doing his best.

Deflating anger and resentment starts with acknowledging your feelings. While it's nearly impossible to think objectively about intense feelings when you're experiencing them, examining the source of your anger after you've cooled down allows you to step back from the emotion and observe it impartially. Think about your trigger points and "hot buttons." If you're angry at someone, try to separate the behavior from the person as you consider the reasons for it. Sometimes we project our anger onto a person who may not deserve it. By removing yourself from the feeling momentarily, your natural compassion will allow you to see the situation from a kinder perspective.

Sometimes it helps to talk it over with a partner or friend who is already more objective. Depending on your situation, it also may be helpful to take an assertive stance that takes your needs into account. Recognize that your feelings are valid. But then work at letting them go and accepting your situation as fully as you can. Recognize and appreciate the positive moments that you would not have had without the difficult ones. Acceptance and gratitude for the silver linings will help to replace anger and resentment with peace.

Inadequacy

It's not uncommon for women struggling with milk production to confide that they feel inadequate as mothers and that their babies deserve better. Yet mothering is not about perfection or proving yourself to anyone; it is about creating relationships. Think about how much your baby is growing to love you and how much you are growing to love him. Many kinds of milk can nurture the body, but only your love can nurture his soul.

Feeling Rejected by Baby

In the midst of all your hard work, it can be dismaying if baby seems more satisfied by the supplement than your milk. Even worse, if he fusses during feeding at the breast, it can feel as if he's rejecting you. Such a belief can profoundly affect the way you feel about yourself as a mother and undermine your confidence. In these moments, it is important to realize that feelings of rejection are an *interpretation* of your baby's feeding behavior, not the *reality* of how your baby feels about you as his mother. Keep in mind that you are his mother, no matter what. You are the person who knows him best. You are the person *he* knows best. You are the person he thinks about when he needs comfort. His need and love for you are deep, even though he cannot yet tell you this in words.

Feeling Selfish for Wanting to Breastfeed

It's ironic that in the midst of the struggle, you may feel or be told that you are being selfish for wanting to breastfeed your baby. But think about your original motives for breastfeeding. You simply want to give your baby the wonderful and normal relationship of feeding him at your breast and the lifelong benefit of the unique nutrition and immunities of human milk. This is not selfish.

Feeling Judgmental of Other Mothers

Some mothers who struggle find it very disturbing to see other mothers overflowing with milk who wean early. The reality is that we can never know what is in the hearts and life experiences of other mothers. Their reasons not to breastfeed or apparent lack of persistence in the face of problems may be related to serious personal issues—present or past—that make breastfeeding as much a difficulty for them as breastfeeding with low milk production is for you. On the other hand, it may be that they simply didn't have accurate information about the benefits and joys of breastfeeding or the support they needed to overcome other obstacles.

Feeling Lonely

Breastfeeding in the face of low milk supply can be difficult and lonely. Support is as important as good information when working on breastfeeding issues. You simply cannot do it all alone. Meeting other mothers who have felt the same way and faced similar challenges is reassuring and validating. They may even have ideas to help that only someone who has experienced similar issues herself could know. If you enjoy the online world, you may find solace in an Internet breastfeeding support group such as Mothers Overcoming Breastfeeding Issues (MOBI) (www.mobimotherhood .org). For those who prefer meeting others in person, there are local support groups like La Leche League throughout the world (see www.llli.org).

Feeling Hurt by Insensitive Remarks and Criticism

One new mother was asked by a nurse how breastfeeding was going. When the mother answered that she was having to supplement, the nurse replied, "Of course you do, dear. Most new moms have to supplement. You'll get it right with the next baby."

Sometimes people say hurtful things even though they mean well. It's similar to wanting to comfort a bereaved person after a death but not knowing quite what to say and uttering something insensitive instead. If firmly held beliefs about infant feeding are being challenged, the person may be especially unable to show empathy. On other occasions, the remarks may even be outright criticisms.

The natural reaction to hurtful comments is defensiveness, usually expressed by an angry reply or stunned silence. However, standing up for yourself doesn't have to mean a full-blown confrontation. Say something that acknowledges the other person's concern without agreeing with it; this tactfully asserts your right to your position. For instance, if Great-Aunt Matilda says that you are wasting away your baby's childhood with "all this breastfeeding nonsense," you can take a deep breath, think about what she might really be concerned about, and calmly reply, "It sounds like you're worried that I'm not spending enough time nurturing and enjoying my baby." Stop there. Don't justify what you are doing. Answer her next comment, which is likely to be a bit gentler, with another simple articulation of her fears. Addressing her underlying concerns may lead to a genuine, respectful discussion that can help you both understand each other better.

It can feel even more hurtful to be criticized by another nursing mother because you're not breastfeeding exclusively. Mothers tell stories about feeling judged by other moms at breastfeeding support group meetings because they were supplementing with formula. Don't wait for the shoe to drop; head off judgment by explaining up front that you have to supplement because you don't have enough milk yet, and that you're there because you need support. Once they understand your situation, they'll almost certainly empathize and applaud your efforts to breastfeed. If not, don't be discouraged. Look for a more accepting group, even if it is farther away. It's worth the effort to find a group that is open-minded and understanding of the challenges you're facing. Fortunately, there are many out there waiting to welcome you. For more ways to cope with criticism about breastfeeding, visit www.kellymom .com/bf/criticism.html and www.llli.org/faq/criticism.html.

Feeling Overwhelmed

The struggle to make more milk, lack of sleep, and never-ending obligations may wear you down until you feel as though you are sinking into an abyss. When you become aware of these feelings, it is time to find a reenergizing activity that can make you feel better without interfering with your breastfeeding efforts. Sneaking off for a bubble bath when dad comes home, for instance, or escaping for a manicure or a quick cup of coffee with a friend can really help recharge your batteries. It is amazing what a few moments of self-pampering and indulgence can do for your outlook. Involving family members to help with things like washing pump parts can also reduce some of the responsibilities that feel overwhelming. If these suggestions don't seem enough, seek help from a baby-friendly therapist who will support your efforts to breastfeed but help you maintain emotional balance.

Feeling Depressed

Most mothers experience some moments of depression when they have a new baby, even when their road is smooth. Exhaustion from adjusting to the nighttime needs of a baby can magnify these feelings. This can also be a normal response to the sudden shift in self-image and identity as a woman becomes a mother and undertakes the great responsibility of parenting. Coping with low milk production puts you at higher risk for depression because you are under additional stress as you do double duty, taking care of baby and working to build your milk supply. Have people begun hinting that you should wean? Don't listen to them. Weaning often leads to increased depression, not less.[1]

In most cases, depression improves when your physical and emotional needs are being met. When was the last time you had enough sleep, exercise, or a balanced meal? When you take the time to attend to your own needs, your outlook on life will be much more positive. But if you find yourself seriously beyond the brink of exhaustion, one good long sleep can really make a difference. Just once, ask someone else to take care of your baby. Then go to bed and sleep until you wake up on your own. You'll be amazed at how much better you feel, and you may even find yourself producing more milk after a good rest. Take your baby with you for a walk outdoors or at a local mall if it's cold or raining. In the meantime, don't hesitate to ask for help with meals or order takeout if the budget allows. Adding EPA and DHA fatty acid supplements to your diet can also help improve feelings of depression.[2] It is also helpful to share your feelings about your experience with a trusted friend, family member, or partner. Other mothers may be the best confidantes because most have felt depressed at one time or another.

If the depression you feel interferes with your ability to function or care for your baby, you may be experiencing postpartum depression (PPD). Tell your physician or midwife how you are feeling so that they can help you. In some cases medications or herbs are helpful, while in others therapy works well. Medication and therapy combined can also be very effective. In most cases, the drugs to treat PPD are compatible with breastfeeding. Most lactation consultants have a copy of *Medications and Mothers' Milk* by Dr. Thomas Hale that can tell you for sure. Also keep in mind that the usually small risk of the drug is even less with a baby who is partially supported with supplements.

For a more in-depth exploration of the wide range of negative feelings mothers experience, read *The Hidden Feelings of Motherhood: Coping with Stress, Depression, and Burnout* by Dr. Kathleen Kendall-Tackett.

Coping Techniques

It is likely that, as a mother with low milk production, you have experienced at least a few of the emotional issues that we have described. Although it is sometimes necessary to consult a physician or professional therapist, the following coping strategies may also be helpful.

Take It One Day at a Time

A single day can seem to go on forever, and you may wonder how you'll ever manage through weeks and months (or even years) of breastfeeding. On days like that, it is hard to believe that the rough spots will one day be behind you. But try to block out all thoughts of the future. It is easier to handle the effort of breastfeeding just for today. It may even help to say to yourself, "I'll breastfeed just for today and wean tomorrow if I want to." Of course, you'll almost never wean the next day (or anytime soon), but knowing that you *can* provides a sense of control that helps you get through the day.

Set Short Goals

Set short but specific goals that you can easily achieve so you can feel good when you accomplish them. For instance, tell yourself that today you are going to give every supplemental bottle in an upright position to minimize the flow rate. That's easy to do, and at the end of the day you can give yourself a pat on the back for accomplishing that goal. Don't skip the congratulations; you deserve it and you need it. Your confidence will build with each goal you reach.

Fast Forward

This is a great tool when you're at your wits' end and completely overwhelmed with stress. Take a deep breath and try to imagine as vividly as possible what things will be like in five, ten, or even twenty years. For instance, when your four-month-old baby has fussed and cried all day and you don't think you can take another minute, picture ten years from now when your child will be an independent, perfectly charming third-grader, capable of heartwarming conversations and the excitement of discovering new interests. As hard as it is to believe today, you really won't remember most of the stress you were feeling when he was four months old. It really will get easier. And all of the time, patience, and love that you gave him will turn out to be a very worthwhile investment.

Confront Painful Feelings

Take some time alone when you can be unobserved for a while. Make yourself comfortable and put a box of tissues by your side. Then allow all the disappointments of your breastfeeding experience to come to the surface. Feel compassion for yourself—you're completely entitled to these feelings. You may even want to pour it all out into a journal. Or you may prefer the shoulder of a trusted friend; healing seems to reach a deeper level when it is shared with others.

When you're ready to leave the painful feelings behind, make a conscious choice to focus on the good memories. In the same way you took time to think about the painful times, now take time to recount the good times. Look for the silver linings of all the benefits you and your baby received and the personal growth you have experienced. They do exist! You may need to go through this catharsis several times before you feel you've come to terms with all the pain and integrated the positive aspects fully into your memories of this unique time.

Once you've processed your feelings, you have only one hurdle left in order to find peace: forgive yourself for anything you regret. You must be kind to yourself and remember that you made the best decisions you could at the time and you had the best intentions. When you have honestly forgiven yourself and others, you can have complete acceptance and soothing peace about the breastfeeding experiences that you leave behind.

Realize That *You* Are a *Successful* Breastfeeding Mother

This is not about how much milk you were able to produce or how long you were able to breastfeed. It is about the commitment you made to give your baby the best start in life and the tremendous effort you put into pursuing that goal. Even if breastfeeding didn't work out quite the way you may have hoped, you undoubtedly shared some special moments that you would not have had otherwise.

Woven through all the information and strategies we've given you in this book are two important messages. One is that each mother must develop a feeding strategy that best meets the needs of her baby, her family, and herself. The second is that you must view your experience with an appreciation of the mothering capabilities you do have, rather than feeling deprived of what you cannot have. It has taken tremendous courage for you to undertake breastfeeding in a difficult situation. You have set the stage to continue to make parenting choices that will help to form a solid foundation for your baby as he develops an understanding of himself and his worth.

CHAPTER 16

What About Next Time?

Many mothers who've had challenges with milk supply wonder, "What about next time . . . will this happen again? Is there anything I can do now to help with the next baby?" While there are no absolutes, we can tell you that most mothers do make more milk with subsequent babies, though how much more depends on individual circumstances. Having had a previous pregnancy and lactation appears to help because you will likely retain a little of the glandular growth and prolactin receptors, helping the milk-making tissue to be more responsive. The time you've spent breastfeeding up to now is laying a foundation for making more milk in the future.

A Proactive Approach

Now that you've read this book, you have a more complete understanding of what happened or is still happening and what, if anything, can change that path. Working with the advantage of hindsight, you see more of the big picture now, and that puts you in a great position to become proactive. If this baby couldn't remove milk well, the next baby will be starting fresh with a clean slate. You'll know what pitfalls to avoid, and if you missed any windows of opportunity, you'll be ready and waiting for those, as well. Whether you are thinking about another baby or already expecting one, a proactive approach will maximize your chances of making more milk the next time around.

Planning for the Next Pregnancy

Now is the time to explore your options, which vary depending on the cause of the problems. For instance, if inverted nipples caused your problems, consider a device such as the Avent Niplette. Or, you might even look into the possibility of nipple release surgery.

Perhaps you didn't think you had hormonal problems but are wondering now. Sometimes lactation difficulties are the first obvious clue that something in your body isn't working right. There are doctors who might tell you, "some mothers just can't breastfeed," but that's like saying, "some mothers just can't get pregnant." You deserve to have a health care professional (possibly a reproductive endocrinologist) who will investigate *why*. Lactation trouble may just be the first symptom of a health problem. These answers are worth pursuing not only for the next baby but for your own long-term health.

Some intriguing case studies suggest that insufficient glandular tissue may not be a permanent condition in every case. The original researchers of PCOS discovered that some of the young women grew breast tissue where little or none was present once their condition was treated and often went on to breastfeed successfully. Early diagnosis and treatment of PCOS or other hormonal issues, especially during the teen years of critical mammary development for future mothers but also before your next pregnancy, may help minimize problems. Metformin, a diabetes medication that is being used successfully to treat PCOS-related problems in many women, may in some cases correct enough underlying imbalances to allow for better mammary development before and during the next pregnancy. Herbs such as chasteberry and saw palmetto, which are sometimes used as natural treatments for PCOS, have reputations for balancing hormones as well as increasing breast tissue and may be useful between babies.

There are other unconventional ideas for hypoplasia that may be worth exploring as well. Some women have experimented with herbs that have "bust-enhancing" reputations, though there is no research to validate whether glandular tissue is truly affected.

Strategies for a Current Pregnancy

New pregnancies bring new opportunities. Most important is making sure, to the best of your ability, that all of your hormones are functioning properly. Conditions such as thyroid dysfunction should be monitored closely throughout and after pregnancy.

If you have PCOS, are you currently being treated? Many women have used metformin to help normalize their hormones in order to get pregnant. As mentioned previously, research shows that continuing metformin during pregnancy decreases the risk of miscarriage, gestational diabetes, pregnancy hypertension, premature delivery, and pregnancy complications in general; some of these are also risk factors for delayed lactation. It may also allow for better breast development. Discuss this with your physician, and refer him to the technical discussions in *Hale and Hartmann's Textbook of Human Lactation*.

Irene's low milk supply with her first baby was attributed to insufficient glandular tissue. She had taken progesterone injections during her initial pregnancy for the first trimester and experienced breast changes but reported that her breasts reverted back once the hormone was stopped. After discussing this with her doctor during her second pregnancy, she was placed on a regimen of both oral and injected progesterone that was maintained through eight months, after which she slowly weaned off of them. Irene's breast changes sustained better this time, and she delightedly reported that after the birth of her second baby, her milk came in well and she didn't need to supplement at all.

If your progesterone has been low, talk to your doctor about the possibility of supplementation. Progesterone treatment to prevent miscarriage traditionally is discontinued after the first trimester, but for improving glandular growth, therapy through most of the pregnancy may be more effective. Additional progesterone before you conceive also may give your body and breasts a running start.

Some women feel that particular galactogogue herbs have been helpful. Alfalfa during pregnancy and goat's rue during the last trimester have both been credited by some mothers with boosting breast growth. One mother, pregnant with her seventh child after a lapse of several years, was not experiencing the same breast changes as before. After consultation with her lactation consultant and physician at thirty-six weeks, she started taking goat's rue and began to experience changes for the first time just a few days later, including leaking colostrum. (As a beneficial side effect, her blood sugar levels dropped, and her gestational diabetes resolved.) After a slow start and an additional month of herbs, she was able to exclusively breastfeed. It must be emphasized that these herbal applications are experimental and not backed by research. If you are interested but don't have expertise in herbs, consult an herbalist, naturopath, or doctor of Chinese medicine for guidance and by all means talk to your pregnancy health care provider before trying anything.

You Never Know

Angie grew up embarrassed of her small, barely A-sized breasts that she described as looking like "a tennis ball in a tube sock." She was dismayed when she didn't experience the pregnancy breast growth she had looked forward to and then, even worse, wasn't able to produce much milk—just 2 to 4 ounces per day. In addition to nursing, she pumped for a few months with her first child and for more than a year with her next. During that second round, her breasts started filling out and grew multiple cup sizes! With her third baby, she took alfalfa during the end of the pregnancy and additional galactogogues after birth. Her breasts continued to fill out, with normal shape and fullness for the first time in her life. Most amazingly, she made over 70 ounces (2 liters) of milk per day at her high point, much more than her baby needed.

Chana had asymmetrical breasts with especially severe hypoplasia on her right side and experienced only slight enlargement with no tenderness during pregnancy. She struggled to make milk for her first baby with the aid of domperidone, supplementing at breast for two years so she could have a breastfeeding relationship. With her second pregnancy, Chana again had slight enlargement and no tenderness. But this time she was diagnosed with hypothyroidism and began thyroid replacement therapy. After the birth, she nursed frequently, used breast compressions, kept baby skin to skin, and pumped after every feeding with a hospital-grade pump. During the second week, she began using goat's rue, domperidone, and Lactation Blend capsules by Vitanica. She ate oatmeal every day and took a daily flaxseed supplement. Within two weeks, she noticed increased veining and enlargement. Although some supplementation was needed at first, she eventually achieved the exclusive breastfeeding relationship she dreamed about. Chana doesn't attribute her success to any one thing in particular because she believes they all worked synergistically, but she does think that pumping and goat's rue had the biggest effect for her.

These intriguing stories suggest that some primary problems can be improved and sometimes even reversed with subsequent babies. You never know—it's always worth a try!

Hope Is on the Horizon

Research in other fields may also help future mothers who have insufficient glandular tissue. Breast cancer research on turning cell growth off and on may eventually lead to therapy for completing interrupted mammary gland development. This same research has already led to another breakthrough: the ability to grow completely new breast tissue in a mouse from a single stem cell. Researchers envision the ability to replace tissue damaged from breast surgery, but it may eventually be used to help mothers produce more milk as well.[1] These and other advances in women's health have the potential to dramatically increase our milk-making capabilities.

Thank You for Sharing Your Journey with Us

The journey through low milk production that you embarked upon at the beginning of this book is undoubtedly an arduous one. We're honored that you took us with you, and we hope that the information in these pages helped you make more milk for your baby. We admire and applaud all your hard work. You're giving a precious gift not only to your own child but to the emotional and physical health of your future grandchildren and their children as well. It's much more than just milk. Breastfeeding is a legacy that transforms the world.

Appendix

Galactogogue Tables

Note: Do not use the information in these tables without first consulting the explanations about appropriate use of galactogogues in Chapter 12.

Ratings

US Federal Drug Administration

GRAS = Generally Regarded As Safe

Humphrey, *The Nursing Mother's Herbal* (see Sources, p. 244)

A = No contraindications, side effects, drug interactions, or pregnancy-related safety issues have been identified. Generally considered safe when used appropriately.

B = May not be appropriate for self-use by some individuals or dyads, or may cause adverse effects if misused. Seek reliable safety and dose information.

C = Moderate potential for toxicity, mainly dose related. Seek an expert herbalist as well as a lactation consultation before using. Consider using safer herbs.

Nice, *Nonprescription Drugs for the Breastfeeding Mother* (see Sources, p. 244)

Y = Usually safe when breastfeeding

Y19 = Usually safe when breastfeeding; monitor infant for potential side effects

American Herbal Products Association's Botanical Safety Handbook (BSH)

Class 1 = Can be safely consumed when used appropriately

Class 2 = Some restrictions apply

Class 2b = Not to be used during pregnancy

Class 2c = Not be used while nursing

TABLE 1 Herbal Galactogogues

Herb	Therapeutic Dose*		Other Reputed Beneficial Qualities	Potential Side Effects	Cautions/Notes	Rating
	Tea**	Tincture	Capsule				

Herb	Tea**	Tincture	Capsule	Other Reputed Beneficial Qualities	Potential Side Effects	Cautions/Notes	Rating
Alfalfa (*Medicago sativa*)	1–2 tbsp leaves steeped in ⅔ cup (150 mL) water; drink 2–4 times per day	0.5–4 mL 3–4 times per day	1–2 capsules 4 times per day	diuretic, mammary stimulation, pituitary support, calcium, iron, nutritive: vitamins A, C, E, K	loose stools, allergenic for some people, seeds may increase risk of sunburn	related to peanut and legume families; avoid if history of lupus or taking immuno-suppressants	GRAS (spice) Humphrey: leaf: A seed: C Nice: Y19 BSH: Class 1
Aniseed or Anise Seed (*Pimpinella anisum*)	1–2 tsp crushed seeds steeped in 1 cup (240 mL) water 10–20 min.; drink 3–6 times a day	3 mL 2–3 times per day		antiflatulent, anticolic, aromatic, estrogenic, milk ejection aid, relaxing	can be allergenic for some people	not the same as star of anise and should not be used interchangeably; not for medicinal use in pregnancy; avoid if allergic to anthole	GRAS (spice) Humphrey: B Nice: Y19 BSH: Class 2b
Ashwagandha Root (*Withania somnifera*)			one 500 mg capsule concentrated extract twice a day	hypotensive, relaxing, stimulates T4 production in mice	none known	abortifacient: not for use during pregnancy	Humphrey: C BSH: Class 2b

| Herb | Therapeutic Dose* | | | Other Reputed Beneficial Qualities | Potential Side Effects | Cautions/Notes | Rating |
	Tea**	Tincture	Capsule				
Black Cohosh Root (*Cimicifuga racemosa*)		1 mL 3 times per day		hypotensive, milk ejection aid, mammary stimulation	possibly allergenic, occasional gastric discomfort	not for use in pregnancy; sources disagree on lactation, but short-term usually OK; avoid large amounts	Humphrey: B BSH: 2b, 2c
Black Seed / Black Cumin (*Nigella sativa*)	1 tsp crushed seeds steeped in 1 cup (240 mL) water 15 min.; drink 4–6 times per day	1 tbsp seed oil daily		antidiabetic, antihistamine, hypotensive, mammary gland stimulation, nutritive	none known	not recommended during pregnancy; contraindicated with bleeding disorder	GRAS (spice) Humphrey: A
Blessed Thistle (*Cnicus benedictus*)	1–2 tsp dried herb steeped in ⅔ cup (150 mL) water; drink 5–6 times per day (bitter)	1–3 mL 2–4 times per day (bitter)	one to three 250–300 mg capsules 3 times per day when combined with fenugreek; up to 6 g if used alone	antidiarrheal, digestive aid, diuretic, hormone balancer	occasionally allergenic; high doses (more than 1 tsp per cup of tea) may cause gastric irritation	not for use during pregnancy	Humphrey: B Nice: Y19 BSH: 2b

*Dosages are suggested starting points; you may need more or less, depending upon your situation.
**Made with boiling water and loose herb unless otherwise noted, or can use premade tea bags.

continued

TABLE 1 Herbal Galactogogues   *continued*

| Herb | Therapeutic Dose* | | | Other Reputed Beneficial Qualities | Potential Side Effects | Cautions/Notes | Rating |
	Tea**	Tincture	Capsule				
Borage (*Borago officinalis*)	N/A	N/A	1–2 gm oil capsules per day	diuretic, enriches milk, high gamma-linolenic acid (GLA), relaxing	loose stools, minor stomach upset	leaves contain small amounts of toxic alkaloids	Humphrey: seed oil: A leaf: C Nice: Y19 BSH: Class 1 (seed oil)
Caraway Seed (*Carum carvi*)	1–2 tsp freshly crushed seeds steeped in 1 cup (240 mL) water, steep 10–15 min.; drink 5–6 times per day	3 mL 3 times per day	¼–½ tsp powder 3 times per day	antianxiety, anti-flatulent, milk ejection aid, relaxing	none known	avoid large amounts of essential oil	GRAS Humphrey: A Nice: Y BSH: Class 1
Chasteberry or Chaste Tree Berry (*Vitex agnus-castus*)	1 tsp ripe berries infused in 1 cup (240 mL) water 10–15 min.; drink 3 times per day (bitter)	0.5–1 mL (1:5 tincture) 3 times per day or up to 5 mL total daily		hormone balancer, mammary gland stimulation, milk ejection aid, pituitary regulation	itching, rash	may counteract effects of metoclopramide and domperidone, birth control pills; conflicting information on pregnancy use; larger amounts decreased prolactin in men; best used with professional advice	Humphrey: B Nice: Y19 BSH: Class 2b, 2d

| Herb | Therapeutic Dose* | | | Other Reputed Beneficial Qualities | Potential Side Effects | Cautions/Notes | Rating |
	Tea**	Tincture	Capsule				
Coriander Seed (*Coriandrum sativum*)	1 heaping tbsp crushed seeds steeped in 1 cup (240 mL) water 10–15 min.; drink 3–5 times per day			antidiabetic, antiflatulent, diuretic; milk ejection aid, nutritive	increased photosensitivity (rare)	related to celery; avoid large amounts	Humphrey: A Nice: Y19 BSH: Class 1
Dandelion Leaves (*Taraxacum officinale*)	1–2 tsp finely chopped or coarsely powdered leaf steeped in 1 cup (240 mL) water; drink 3 times daily	3 mL 3 times per day	two 500 mg capsules 3 times per day	antidiabetic, diuretic, iron, thyroid support	contact dermatitis (rare)	avoid harvesting from lawns or areas treated with chemicals or pesticides	GRAS (oil, extract) Humphrey: A Nice: Y19 BSH: Class 1
Dill Seed (*Anethum graveolens*)	2 tsp crushed seeds steeped in 1 cup (240 mL) water for 10–15 min.; drink 2–3 times per day	2.5–5 mL 1–3 times per day		antidiabetic, antiflatulent, diuretic, milk ejection aid, relaxing	none known	none known	Humphrey: A Nice: Y BSH: Class 1

*Dosages are suggested starting points; you may need more or less, depending upon your situation.
**Made with boiling water and loose herb unless otherwise noted, or can use premade tea bags.

continued

239

TABLE 1 Herbal Galactogogues *continued*

| Herb | Therapeutic Dose* | | | Other Reputed Beneficial Qualities | Potential Side Effects | Cautions/Notes | Rating |
	Tea**	Tincture	Capsule				
Fennel Seed (*Foeniculum volgare*)	1–3 tsp crushed seeds steeped in 1 cup (240 mL) water 10–15 min.; drink 2–6 times per day	3 mL 3 times per day		antiandrogen, antiflatulent, aromatic, diuretic, estrogenic, hypotensive, mammary gland stimulation, milk ejection aid, relaxing	contact dermatitis	related to celery; essential oil may be toxic in very large amounts; avoid essential oil during pregnancy	GRAS (spice) Humphrey: A Nice: Y19 BSH: Class 1
Fenugreek Seed (*Trigonella foenum-graecum*)	1 tsp whole or ¼ tsp powdered seeds steeped in 1 cup (240 mL) water 15 min.; drink 2–3 times per day	1–2 mL 3 times per day	one to four 580–610 mg capsules 3–4 times per day or equivalent	antidiabetic, hypotensive, iron, mammary gland stimulation	can cause maple syrup smell in mother or baby, stomach upset, loose stools/diarrhea, hypoglycemia; powdered seed form may cause allergic reactions, especially in asthmatics	consult physician first if history of hypoglycemia or diabetes; take with food to minimize hypoglycemic effects; reduces thyroid T3 in mice and rats; not for use during pregnancy; avoid fenugreek-thyme combinations; seeds have high mucilage content; don't take with medications (tincture OK)	GRAS (spice) Humphrey: B Nice: Y19 BSH: 2b

Herb	Therapeutic Dose*			Other Reputed Beneficial Qualities	Potential Side Effects	Cautions/Notes	Rating
	Tea**	Tincture	Capsule				
Goat's Rue (*Galega Officinalis*)	1 tsp leaves steeped in 1 cup (240 mL) water for 10–15 min.; drink 2–5 times per day (bitter)	Wise Woman Herbals: 2.5 mL 1–4 times per day; Turner: 3–4 mL 4 times per day; Motherlove: 1–2 mL 4 times per day; Dr. Low Dog: 1 tsp (5 mL) in 8 oz (240 mL) water 3 times per day	Motherlove: one capsule 4 times per day, or two capsules 3 times per day for over 175 lb	antidiabetic, diuretic, mammary gland stimulation	hypoglycemic, may have blood-thinning properties	consult with health care provider if taking any other diabetic-related medications; take with food to reduce any hypoglycemic effects; observe for hypoglycemia if taken together with antidiabetic medications such as metformin; no research regarding pregnancy	Humphrey: B Nice: Y
Hops Flower (*Humulus lupulus*)	1 tsp leaves steeped in 1 cup (240 mL) water 10 min.; drink 1–2 times per day		two 350 mg capsules 3 times per day	mammary gland stimulation, milk ejection aid	contact allergy	use with history of depression controversial	GRAS (oil, extract) Humphrey: B BSH: 2d

*Dosages are suggested starting points; you may need more or less, depending upon your situation.
**Made with boiling water and loose herb unless otherwise noted, or can use premade tea bags.

continued

TABLE 1 Herbal Galactogogues *continued*

Herb	Therapeutic Dose*			Other Reputed Beneficial Qualities	Potential Side Effects	Cautions/Notes	Rating
	Tea**	Tincture	Capsule				
Marshmallow Root (*Althaea officinalis*)	1 tbsp root powder in 5–8 oz (150–140 mL) cold water, let stand 30 min.; drink immediately	1–4 mL 3 times per day	two to four capsules 3 times per day	diuretic, enriches milk, nutritive: vitamin A, calcium, zinc, iron, sodium, iodine, and B-complex vitamins	allergic reactions possible, but extremely rare	high mucilage content; avoid taking medications at same time	Humphrey: A Nice: Y19 BSH: Class 1
Milk Thistle (*Silybum marianum*)	1 heaping tsp freshly crushed/ chopped seeds steeped in 5 oz (150 mL) water 20–30 min.; drink up to 5–6 times per day	3–5 mL 3 times per day	two 500 mg standardized capsules 3 times per day	antidiabetic, liver and gallbladder protective	possible allergen, possible mild laxative effect in first few days	take with food if any hypoglycemic effects; may reduce effectiveness of metronidazole	Humphrey: A Nice: Y19 BSH: Class 1
Nettle or Stinging Nettle (*Urtica urens* or *Urtica dioica*)	1 tbsp cut herb steeped in 1 cup (240 mL) water for 10–15 min.; drink 2–3 times per day	2.5–5 mL (½–1 tsp) leaf tincture 3 times per day	one to two 300 mg capsule 3 times per day	antidiabetic, antiinflammatory, diuretic, hypotensive, nutritive: iron, calcium, vitamin K, potassium	mild diuretic, mild gastrointestinal upset	none known	Humphrey: A BSH: Class 1

| Herb | Therapeutic Dose* | | | Other Reputed Beneficial Qualities | Potential Side Effects | Cautions/Notes | Rating |
	Tea**	Tincture	Capsule				
Oat Straw/ Oats (*Avena sativa*)	1 tbsp dried oat straw steeped in 1 cup (240 mL) water 10–15 min.; drink 3 times per day	3–5 mL 3 times per day	two 600–700 mg capsules 2–3 times per day	antidepressant, antianxiety, diuretic, pituitary support, nutritive: iron, magnesium	none known	avoid with celiac disease (contains gluten)	Humphrey: A Nice: Y BSH: Class 1
Red Clover (*Trifolium pratense*)	1–3 tsp herb steeped in 1 cup water 10–15 min.; drink 3 times per day	2–6 mL 3 times per day	two to three capsules 3 times per day	diuretic, mammary gland stimulation, nutritive, increases thyroid hormone in ewes	rarely may cause loose stools or nausea	*avoid fermented red clover*; avoid taking with blood thinners, aspirin or hormonal birth control; use during pregnancy controversial though moderate amounts probably fine; usually taken with other herbs	GRAS (spice, oil) Humphrey: B Nice: Y BSH: 2b
Red Raspberry Leaf (*Rubus idaeus*)	1 tsp steeped in ⅔ cup (150 mL) water 5 min.; drink 2–4 times per day	3–4 mL 3 times per day	three 300 mg capsules 3 times per day	milk ejection aid, nutritive: iron, calcium	none known	some sources believe it may cause lowering of milk production with long-term use (more than 2 weeks)	Humphrey: A Nice: Y19 BSH: Class 1

*Dosages are suggested starting points; you may need more or less, depending upon your situation.
**Made with boiling water and loose herb unless otherwise noted, or can use premade tea bags.

continued

TABLE 1 Herbal Galactogogues *continued*

| Herb | Therapeutic Dose* | | | Other Reputed Beneficial Qualities | Potential Side Effects | Cautions/Notes | Rating |
	Tea**	Tincture	Capsule				
Saw Palmetto (*Serenoa repens*)	½–1 tsp berries in 1 cup (240 mL) water, bring to a boil and simmer gently for 5 min.; drink 3 times per day	1–2 mL 3 times per day	one to two capsules powdered berries 2–3 times per day	antiandrogen, diuretic, hormone balancer, mammary gland stimulation	occasional stomach upset, diarrhea, headache, take with food to avoid	avoid with bleeding disorder	Humphrey: A BSH: Class 1
Shatavari (*Asparagus racemosus*)	powder: 2 tsp stirred into warm milk 1–2 times a day		one to two 500 mg capsules concentrated extract 2 times per day	diuretic, mammary gland stimulation, nutritive	may have laxative effect	not recommended during pregnancy	Humphrey: B
Vervain (*Verbena officinalis*)	1 tsp steeped in ⅔ cup (150 mL) water 10 min.; drink 3 times per day; or ¼–½ cup herb in 1 qt (1 L) water 10–15 min.; drink ½ cup 3 times per day	2–4 mL 3 times per day		antianxiety, hypotensive, thyroid support	none known	usually combined with other herbs rather than taken alone; not recommended during pregnancy	GRAS (flavoring) Humphrey: B Nice: Y BSH: 2b

*Dosages are suggested starting points; you may need more or less, depending upon your situation.

**Made with boiling water and loose herb unless otherwise noted, or can use premade tea bags.

Sources: See Chapter 12 citations in References. In addition: Humphrey S. *The Nursing Mother's Herbal.* Minneapolis, MN: Fairview Press; 2003. Nice, F. *Nonprescription Drugs for the Breastfeeding Mother.* Amarillo, TX: Hale Publishing; 2007. McGuffin M, Hobbs C, Upton R, Goldberg A, eds. *American Herbal Products Association Botanical Safety Handbook.* Boca Raton, FL: CRC Press; 1997. Wise Woman Herbals; www.wisewomanherbals.com. Mechell Turner; www.birthandbreastfeeding.com. Motherlove Herbal Company; www.motherlove.com. Dr. Low Dog; www.drlowdog.com.

TABLE 2 Symptoms and Herbs That May Be Beneficial to Them

Symptom	Herbal Properties	Herbs
heavy bleeding, hemorrhage, anemia	high iron content or pituitary support	alfalfa, nettle, red raspberry, oat straw, fenugreek, dandelion
hypertension (high blood pressure)	hypotensive	fennel, fenugreek, nettle, vervain, black cohosh, ashwagandha, black seed
postpartum edema (water retention)	diuretic	alfalfa, blessed thistle, borage, coriander, dandelion, dill, fennel, goat's rue, nettle, oat straw, red clover, saw palmetto, shatavari, marshmallow
stress	relaxing aromatic herbs	anise, caraway, dill, fennel
maternal or infant gassiness	antiflatulent (gas) carminatives	anise, caraway, dill, fennel, hops
slow milk ejection	increase flow of milk or relaxing to help milk flow	anise, black cohosh, caraway, chasteberry, coriander, dill, fennel, red raspberry, wild lettuce (Lactuca virosa)
history of high blood sugar or insulin resistance	antidiabetic (check with your physician also)	fenugreek, coriander, goat's rue, nettle, dandelion, milk thistle, black seed
hormonal imbalances	hormone balancer	blessed thistle, chasteberry, saw palmetto
hyperandrogenism	antiandrogen (male hormone)	saw palmetto, fennel
hypothyroid	thyroid-supporting qualities	ashwagandha, dandelion, nettle, vervain, red clover
hyperthyroid	anti-thyroid	fenugreek
mammary hypoplasia or poor pregnancy breast development	mammary gland stimulation (often estrogenic)	goat's rue, chasteberry, fennel, fenugreek, red clover, saw palmetto, shatavari, alfalfa, black seed, black cohosh, hops

TABLE 3 Selected Lactogenic Homeopathic Remedies for Low Milk Supply

For best results, consult with a homeopathic practitioner.

Homeopathic Remedy	Clinical Indication
Agnus castus	depression
Calcarea carbonica	general use; hemorrhage or anemia
Causticum	short-term exhaustion; works best with personality that resists rather than "rolls with the punches"
Dulcamara	sudden loss of milk after exposure to cold and damp; engorgement
Galega	anemia or poor nutrition
Helonias	extreme maternal exhaustion (supermom syndrome)
Ignatia	sudden loss of milk related to shock and grief
Lactuca virosa	strong; general use
Ricinus communis	hemorrhage or anemia
Urtica urens	general use; hemorrhage or anemia

Source: Hatherly P. *The Homeopathic Physician's Guide to Lactation*. Brisbane, Australia: Luminoz Pty Ltd; 2004; www.patriciahatherly.com/book.html.

References

Chapter 1

1. Kent J, Mitoulas L, Cregan M, Ramsay D, Doherty D, Hartmann P. Volume and frequency of breastfeedings and fat content of breast milk throughout the day. *Pediatrics*. 2006;e117(3):387–95.

2. DeCarvalho M, Robertson S, Friedman A, Klaus M. Effect of frequent breast-feeding on early milk production and infant weight gain. *Pediatrics*. 1983;72(3):307–11.

Theil P, Seirsen K, Hurley W, Labouriau R, Thomsen B, Sørensen M. Role of suckling in regulating cell turnover and onset and maintenance of lactation in individual mammary glands of sows. *J Anim Sci*. 2006;84(7):1691–8.

Kim J, Mizoguchi Y, Yamaguchi H, Enami J, Sakai S. Removal of milk by suckling acutely increases the prolactin receptor gene expression in the lactating mouse mammary gland. *Mol Cell Endocrinol*. 1997;131(1):31–8.

3. Kent J, Mitoulas L, Cregan M, Ramsay D, Doherty D, Hartmann P. Volume and frequency of breastfeedings and fat content of breast milk throughout the day. *Pediatrics*. 2006;117(3):387–95.

4. Vetharaniam I, Davis S, Soboleva T, Shorten P, Wake G. Modeling the interaction of milking frequency and nutrition on mammary gland growth and lactation. *J Dairy Sci*. 2003;86(6):1987–96.

5. Daly S, Owens R, Hartmann P. The short-term synthesis and infant-regulated removal of milk in lactating women. *Exp Physiol.* 1993;78:209–20.

Kent J, Mitoulas L, Cregan M, Ramsay D, Doherty D, Hartmann P. Volume and frequency of breastfeedings and fat content of breast milk throughout the day. *Pediatrics.* 2006;117(3):e387–95.

6. Woolridge M. Problems of establishing lactation. *Food Nutr Bull.* 1996;17(4):316–23.

Chapter 2

1. Cox D, Owens R, Hartmann P. Blood and milk prolactin and the rate of milk synthesis in women. *Exp Physiol.* 1996;81(6):1007–20.

2. Cregan M, Mitoulas L, Hartmann P. Milk prolactin, feed volume and duration between feeds in women breastfeeding their full-term infants over a 24 h period. *Exp Physiol.* 2002;87(2):207–14.

3. Kent J, Mitoulas L, Cregan M, Ramsay D, Doherty D, Hartmann P. Volume and frequency of breastfeedings and fat content of breast milk throughout the day. *Pediatrics.* 2006;117(3):e387–95.

4. Cregan M, Mitoulas L, Hartmann P. Milk prolactin, feed volume and duration between feeds in women breastfeeding their full-term infants over a 24 h period. *Exp Physiol.* 2002;87(2):207–14.

5. Dewey K, Heinig J, Nommsen L, Lonnerdal B. Maternal versus infant factors related to breast milk intake and residual milk volume: the DARLING study. *Pediatrics.* 1991;87(6):829–37.

Chapter 3

1. Scanlon K, Alexander M, Serdula M, Davis M, Bowman B. Assessment of infant feeding: the validity of measuring milk intake. *Nutr Rev.* 2002;60(8):235–51.

2. Lai C, Hale T, Kent J, Simmer K, Hartmann P. Hourly rate of milk synthesis in women. Paper presented at: the 12th International Conference of the International Society for Research into Human Milk and Lactation (ISRHML); September 10–14, 2004; Cambridge, England.

Chapter 4

1. Israel-Ballard K, Coutsoudis A, Chantry C, et al. Bacterial safety of flash-heated and unheated expressed breastmilk during storage. *J Trop Pediatr.* 2006;52(6):399–405.

Jeffery B, Webber L, Mokhondo K, Erasmus D. Determination of the effectiveness of inactivation of human immunodeficiency virus by Pretoria pasteurization. *J Trop Pediatr.* 2001;47(6):345–9.

2. Smith W, Erenberg A, Nowak A. Imaging evaluation of the human nipple during breast-feeding. *Am J Dis Child.* 1988;142:76–8.

Chapter 5

1. Cox S. Expressing and storing colostrum antenatally for use in the newborn period. *Breastfeed Rev.* 2006;14(3):11–16.

2. Moscone S, Moore M. Breastfeeding during pregnancy. *J Hum Lact.* 1993;9(2):83–8.

Merchant K, Martorell R, Haas J. Maternal and fetal responses to the stresses of lactation concurrent with pregnancy and of short recuperative intervals. *Am J Clin Nutr.* 1990;52(2):280–8.

3. Righard L, Alade M. Effect of delivery room routines on success of first breast-feed. *Lancet.* 1990;336(8723):1105–7.

4. Kroeger M, Smith L. *Impact of Birthing Practices on Breastfeeding: Protecting the Mother and Baby Continuum.* Sudbury, MA: Jones and Bartlett Publishers; 2004.

Baumgarder D, Muehl P, Fischer M, Pribbenow B. Effect of labor epidural anesthesia on breast-feeding of healthy full-term newborns delivered vaginally. *J Am Board Fam Pract*. 2003;16(1):7–13.

Jordan S, Emery S, Bradshaw C, Watkins A, Friswell W. The impact of intrapartum analgesia on infant feeding. *BJOG*. 2005;112(7):927–34.

5. Dewey K, Nommsen-Rivers L, Heinig M, Cohen R. Risk factors for suboptimal infant breastfeeding behavior, delayed onset of lactation, and excess neonatal weight loss. *Pediatrics*. 2003;112(3 Pt 1):607–19.

Grajeda R, Pérez-Escamilla R. Stress during labor and delivery is associated with delayed onset of lactation among urban Guatemalan women. *J Nutr*. 2002;132(10):3055–60.

Rowe-Murray H, Fisher J. Baby friendly hospital practices: cesarean section is a persistent barrier to early initiation of breastfeeding. *Birth*. 2002;29(2):124–31.

6. Hurst N, Valentine C, Renfro L, Burns P, Ferlic L. Skin-to-skin holding in the neonatal intensive care unit influences maternal milk volume. *J Perinatol*. 1997;17(3):213–7.

7. Varendi H, Porter R, Winberg J. Attractiveness of amniontic fluid odor: evidence of prenatal olfactory learning? *Acta Paediatr*. 1996;85(10):1223–7.

Varendi H, Porter R, Winberg J. Natural odour preferences of newborn infants change over time. *Acta Paediatr*. 1997;86(9):985–90.

8. Jones E, Dimmock P, Spencer S. A randomised controlled trial to compare methods of milk expression after preterm delivery. *Arch Dis Child Fetal Neonatal Ed*. 2001;85(2):F91–5.

9. Freeman M, Kanyicska B, Lerant A, Nagy G. Prolactin: structure, function, and regulation of secretion. *Physiol Rev*. 2000;80(4):1523–631.

Stern J, Reichlin S. Prolactin circadian rhythm persists throughout lactation in women. *Neuroendocrin*. 1990;51(1):31–7.

Chapter 6

1. Aljazaf K, Hale T, Ilett K, et al. Pseudoephedrine: effects on milk production in women and estimation of infant exposure via breastmilk. *Br J Clin Pharmacol.* 2003;56(1):18–24.

2. Koletzko B, Lehner F. Beer and breastfeeding. *Adv Exp Med Biol.* 2000;478:23–8.

Mennella J. Short-term effects of maternal alcohol consumption on lactational performance. *Alcohol Clin Exp Res.* 1998;22(7):1389–92.

Mennella J, Pepino M, Teff K. Acute alcohol consumption disrupts the hormonal milieu of lactating women. *J Clin Endocrinol Metab.* 2005;90(4):1979–85.

3. Andersen A, Lund-Andersen C, Larsen J, et al. Suppressed prolactin but normal neurophysin levels in cigarette smoking breastfeeding women. *Clin Endocrinol (Oxf).* 1982;17(4):363–8.

Hopkinson J, Schanler R, Fraley J, Garza C. Milk production by mothers of premature infants: influence of cigarette smoking. *Pediatrics.* 1992;90(6):934–8.

4. Moscone S, Moore J. Breastfeeding during pregnancy. *J Hum Lact.* 1993;9(2):83–8.

5. Hartmann P. Personal communication with Lisa Marasco. December 19, 2004.

6. Gartner L. Hyperbilirubinemia and breastfeeding. In: Hale T, Hartmann P, eds. *Hale & Hartmann's Textbook of Human Lactation.* Amarillo, TX: Hale Publishing; 2007:255–70.

7. Howard C, Howard F, Lanphear B, de Blieck E, Eberly S, Lawrence R. The effects of early pacifier use on breastfeeding duration. *Pediatrics.* 1999;103(3):E33.

Mitchell E, Blair P, L'Hoir M. Should pacifiers be recommended to prevent sudden infant death syndrome? *Pediatrics.* 2006;117(5):1755–8.

McKenna J, McDade T. Why babies should never sleep alone: a review of the co-sleeping controversy in relation to SIDS, bed-sharing and breastfeeding. *Paediatr Respir Rev.* 2005;6(2);134–52.

8. Ezzo G, Bucknam R. *On Becoming Babywise.* Simi Valley, CA: Parent-Wise Solutions, Inc.; 2006.

9. Berger K. *The Developing Person Through Childhood and Adolescence.* 6th ed. New York: Worth Publishers; 2003.

10. Marasco L, Barger J. Cue vs. scheduled feeding: revisiting the controversy. *Mother Baby J.* 1998;3(4):39–42.

11. Lunn P, Prentice A, Austin S, Whitehead R. Influence of maternal diet on plasma-prolactin levels during lactation. *Lancet.* 1980;1(8169):623–5.

Smith C. Effects of maternal undernutrition upon the newborn infant in Holland (1944–1945). *J Pediatr.* 1947;30(3):229–43.

12. Butte N, Garza C, Stuff J, Smith E, Nichols B. Effect of maternal diet and body composition on lactational performance. *Am J Clin Nutr.* 1984;39(2):296–306.

Strode M, Dewey K, Lönnerdal B. Effects of short-term caloric restriction on lactational performance of well-nourished women. *Acta Paediatr Scand.* 1986;75(2):222–9.

13. Bowles B, Williamson B. Pregnancy and lactation following anorexia and bulimia. *J Obstet Gynecol Neonatal Nurs.* 1990;19(3):243–8.

Monteleone P, Brambilla F, Bortolotti F, Ferraro C, Maj M. Plasma prolactin response to D-fenfluramine is blunted in bulimic patients with frequent binge episodes. *Psychol Med.* 1998;28(4):975–83.

14. Kuhne T, Bubl R, Baumgartner R. Maternal vegan diet causing a serious infantile neurological disorder due to vitamin B_{12} deficiency. *Eur J Pediatr.* 1991;150(3):205–8.

15. Fussy S. The skinny on gastric by-pass: what pharmacists need to know. *US Pharm.* 2005;2:HS-3–12.

16. Ferraro D. Management of the bariatric surgery patient: lifelong postoperative care (Board Review). *Clinician Reviews.* 2004;14(2):73–80.

17. Dailey A. Personal communication with Lisa Marasco. August 12, 2004.

18. Olsen A. Nursing under conditions of thirst or excessive ingestion of fluids. *Acta Obstet et Gynecol.* 1939;10(4):312–43.

19. Dusdieker L, Booth B, Stumbo P, Eichenberger J. Effect of supplemental fluids on human milk production. *J Pediatr.* 1985;106(2):207–11.

Chapter 7

1. Bahr D. *Oral Motor Assessment and Treatment: Ages and Stages.* Needham Heights, MA: Allyn and Bacon; 2001.

2. Vallone S. Chiropractic evaluation and treatment of musculo-skeletal dysfunction in infants demonstrating difficulty breastfeeding. *J Clin Chiro Ped.* 2004;5(1):349–61.

3. Brussel C. Craniosacral therapy in difficult situations. *Leaven.* 2001;37(4) 82–3.

4. Ballard J, Auer C, Khoury J. Ankyloglossia: assessment, incidence, and effect of frenuloplasty on the breastfeeding dyad. *Pediatrics.* 2002;110(5):e63.

Kupietzky A, Botzer E. Ankyloglossia in the infant and young child: clinical suggestions for diagnosis and management. *Pediatr Dent.* 2005;27(1):40–6.

Ricke L, Baker N, Madlon-Kay D, DeFor T. Newborn tongue-tie: prevalence and effect on breast-feeding. *J Am Board Fam Pract.* 2005;18(1):1–7.

Messner A, Lalakea M, Aby J, Macmahon J, Bair E. Ankyloglossia: incidence and associated feeding difficulties. *Arch Otolaryngol Head Neck Surg.* 2000;126(1):36–9.

5. Watson Genna C, ed. *Supporting Sucking Skills in Breastfeeding Infants*. Sudbury, MA: Jones and Bartlett Publishers; 2008.

6. Amir L, James J, Beatty J. Review of tongue-tie release at a tertiary maternity hospital. *J Paediatr Child Health*. 2005;41(5–6): 243–5.

Dollberg S, Botzer E, Grunis E, Mimouni F. Immediate nipple pain relief after frenotomy in breast-fed infants with ankyloglossia: a randomized, prospective study. *J Pediatr* Surg. 2006;41(9):1598–600.

Hogan M, Westcott C, Griffiths M. Randomized, controlled trial of division of tongue-tie infants with feeding problems. *J Paediatr Child Health*. 2005;41(5–6):246–50.

Srinivasan A, Dobrich C, Mitnick H, Feldman P. Ankyloglossia in breastfeeding infants: the effect of frenotomy on maternal nipple pain and latch. *Breastfeed Med*. 2006;1(4):216–24.

7. Messner A, Lalakea M. The effect of ankyloglossia on speech in children. *Otolaryngol Head Neck Surg*. 2002;127(6):539–45.

Lalakea M, Messner A. Ankyloglossia: the adolescent and adult perspective. *Otolaryngol Head Neck Surg*. 2003;128(5):746–52.

8. Watson Genna C, ed. *Supporting Sucking Skills in Breastfeeding Infants*. Sudbury, MA: Jones and Bartlett Publishers; 2008.

9. Lambert J, Watters N. Breastfeeding the infant/child with a cardiac defect: an informal survey. *J Hum Lact*. 1998;14(2):151–5.

Marino B, O'Brien P, LoRe H. Oxygen saturations during breast and bottle feedings in infants with congenital heart disease. *J Pediatr Nurs*. 1995;10(6):360–4.

10. Weiss-Salinas D, Williams N. Sensory defensiveness: a theory of its effect on breastfeeding. *J Hum Lact*. 2001;17(2):145–51.

Chapter 8

1. Dewey K, Nommsen-Rivers L, Heinig M, Cohen R. Risk factors for suboptimal infant breastfeeding behavior, delayed onset of lactation, and excess neonatal weight loss. *Pediatrics.* 2003; 112(3 Pt 1):607–19.

2. Han S, Hong Y. The inverted nipple: its grading and surgical correction. *Plast Reconstr Surg.* 1999;104(2):389–95.

3. McGeorge D. The "Niplette": an instrument for the non-surgical correction of inverted nipples. *Br J Plast Surg.* 1994;47(1):46–9.

Ozcan M, Kahveci R. The "Niplette" for the non-surgical correction of inverted nipples. *Br J Plast Surg.* 1995;48(2):115.

4. Neifert M, Seacat J, Jobe W. Lactation failure due to insufficient glandular development of the breast. *Pediatrics.* 1985;76(5): 823–28.

Huggins K, Petok E, Mireles O. Markers of lactation insufficiency: a study of 34 mothers. *Current Issues in Clinical Lactation.* 2000:25–35.

5. Markey C, Rubin B, Soto A, Sonnenschein C. Endocrine disruptors: from wingspread to environmental developmental biology. *Steroid Biochem Mol Biol.* 2003;83(1–5):235–44.

6. Fenton S, Hamm J, Birnbaum L, Youngblood G. Persistent abnormalities in the rat mammary gland following gestational and lactational exposure to 2,3,7,8-tetrachlorodibenzo-p-dioxin (TCDD). *Toxicol Sci.* 2002;67(1):63–74.

Gladen B, Rogan W. DDE and shortened duration of lactation in a northern Mexican town. *Am J Public Health.* 1995;85(4):504–8.

Guillette E, Conard C, Lares F, Aguilar M, McLachlan J, Guillette L. Altered breast development in young girls from an agricultural environment. *Environ Health Perspect.* 2006;114(3):471–5.

7. Huggins K, Petok E, Mireles O. Markers of lactation insufficiency: a study of 34 mothers. *Current Issues in Clinical Lactation.* 2000:25–35.

8. Ramsay D, Kent J, Hartmann R, Hartmann P. Anatomy of the lactating human breast redefined with ultrasound imaging. *J Anat.* 2005;206(6):525–34.

9. Schlenz I, Kuzbari R, Gruber H, Holle J. The sensitivity of the nipple-areola complex: an anatomic study. *Plast Reconstr Surg.* 2000;105(3):905–9.

10. Deutinger M, Domanig E. Breast development and areola sensitivity after submammary skin incision for median sternotomy. *Ann Thorac Surg.* 1992;53(6):1023–4.

11. Mofid M, Klatsky S, Singh N, Nahabedian M. Nipple-areola complex sensitivity after primary breast augmentation: a comparison of periareolar and inframammary incision approaches. *Plast Reconstr Surg.* 2006;117(6):1694–8.

12. Michalopoulos K. The effects of breast augmentation surgery on future ability to lactate. *Breast J.* 2007;13(1):62–7.

13. Souto G, Giugliani E, Giugliani C, Schneider M. The impact of breast reduction surgery on breastfeeding performance. *J Hum Lact.* 2003;19(1):43–9.

14. Slien W, Matory W, Love S. *Atlas of Techniques in Breast Surgery.* Phildelphia/New York: Lippincott-Raven; 1996:18–9.

15. Halbert L. Breastfeeding in the woman with a compromised nervous system. *J Hum Lact.* 1998;14(4):327–31.

16. Cowley K. Psychogenic and pharmacologic induction of the let-down reflex can facilitate breastfeeding by tetraplegic women: a report of 3 cases. *Arch Phys Med Rehabil.* 2005;86:1261–4.

Chapter 9

1. Saito T, Tojo K, Oki Y, et al. A case of prolactin deficiency with familial puerperal alactogenesis accompanying impaired ACTH secretion. *Endocr J.* 2007;54(1):59–62.

2. Zargar A, Salahuddin M, Laway B, Masoodi S, Ganie M, Bhat M. Puerperal alactogenesis with normal prolactin dynamics: is prolactin resistance the cause? *Fertil Steril.* 2000;74(3):598–600.

3. Rasmussen K, Kjolhede L. Prepregnant overweight and obesity diminish the prolactin response to suckling in the first week postpartum. *Pediatrics*. 2004;113(5):e465–71.

Rasmussen K. Association of maternal obesity before conception with poor lactation performance. *Annu Rev Nutr*. 2007;27:103–21.

4. Hartmann P, Cregan M. Lactogenesis and the effects of insulin-dependent diabetes mellitus and prematurity. *J Nutr*. 2001;131(11):3016S–20S.

5. Gabbay M. Personal communication with Lisa Marasco. January 28, 2005.

6. Neifert M, DeMarzo S, Seacat J, Young D, Leff M, Orleans M. Influence of breast surgery, breast appearance, and pregnancy-induced breast changes on lactation sufficiency as measured by infant weight gain. *Birth*. 1990;17(1):31–8.

7. Seely E, Maxwell C. Chronic hypertension in pregnancy. *Circulation*. 2007;115(7):e188–90.

8. Henly S, Anderson C, Avery M, Hills-Bonuyk S, Potter S, Duckett L. Anemia and insufficient milk in first-time mothers. *Birth*. 1995;22(2):87–92.

Toppare M, Kitapci F, Senses D, Kaya I, Dilmen U, Laleli Y. Lactational failure-study of risk factors in Turkish mothers. *Indian J Pediatr*. 1994;61(3):269–76.

Rioux F, Savoie N, Allard J. Is there a link between postpartum anemia and discontinuation of breastfeeding? *Can J Diet Pract Res*. 2006;67(2):72–6.

9. Sert M, Tetiker T, Kirim S, Kocak M. Clinical report of 28 patients with Sheehan's syndrome. *Endocr J*. 2003;50(3):297–301.

Willis C, Livingstone V. Infant insufficient milk syndrome associated with maternal postpartum hemorrhage. *J Hum Lact*. 1995;11(2):123–6.

10. O'Dowd R, Kent J, Moseley J, Wlodek M. Effects of utero-placental insufficiency and reducing litter size on maternal mammary function and postnatal offspring growth. *Am J Physiol Regul Integr Comp Physiol.* 2008;294(2):R539–48.

11. Marasco L. The impact of thyroid dysfunction on lactation. *Breastfeeding Abstracts.* 2006;25(2):9, 11–12.

12. Hapon M, Simoncini M, Via G, Jahn G. Effect of hypothyroidism on hormone profiles in virgin, pregnant and lactating rats, and on lactation. *Reproduction.* 2003;126(3):371–82.

Hapon M, Varas S, Jahn G, Giménez M. Effects of hypothyroidism on mammary and liver lipid metabolism in virgin and late-pregnant rats. *J Lipid Res.* 2005;46:1320–30.

13. Rosato R, Giménez M, Jahn G. Effects of chronic thyroid hormone administration on pregnancy, lactogenesis and lactation in the rat. *Acta Endocrinol (Copenh).* 1992;127(6):547–54.

Varas S, Jahn G, Giménez M. Hyperthyroidism affects lipid metabolism in lactating and suckling rats. *Lipids.* 2001; 36(8):801–6.

14. Mandel S, Spencer C, Hollowell J. Are detection and treatment of thyroid insufficiency in pregnancy feasible? *Thyroid.* 2005;15(1):44–53.

15. Lao T. Management of hyperthyroidism and goitre in pregnancy, and postpartum thyroiditis. *Journal of Paediatrics, Obstetrics and Gynaecology.* 2005;31(4):155–64.

16. Sridhar G, Nagamani G. Hypothyroidism presenting with polycystic ovary syndrome. *J Assoc Physicians India.* 1993;41(2):88–90.

17. Marasco L, Marmet C, Shell E. Polycystic ovary syndrome: a connection to insufficient milk supply? *J Hum Lact.* 2000;16(2):143–8.

18. Stein I. Bilateral polycystic ovaries. *Am J Obstet Gynecol.* 1945;50:385–96.

Balcar V, Silinková-Malková E, Matys Z. Soft tissue radiography of the female breast and pelvic pneumoperitoneum in the

Stein-Leventhal syndrome. *Acta Radiol Diagn (Stockh)*. 1972;12(3): 353–62.

19. Thatcher S, Jackson E. Pregnancy outcome in infertile patients with polycystic ovary syndrome who were treated with metformin. *Fertil Steril*. 2006;85(4):1002–9.

20. Vanky E, Isaksen H, Moen M, Carlsen S. Breastfeeding in polycystic ovary syndrome. *Acta Obstet Gynecol Scan*. 2008;87(5):531–5.

21. Baillargeon J, Jakubowicz D, Iuorno M, Jakubowicz S, Nestler J. Effects of metformin and rosiglitazone, alone and in combination, in nonobese women with polycystic ovary syndrome and normal indices of insulin sensitivity. *Fertil Steril*. 2004;82(4):893–902.

22. Glueck C, Wang P, Goldenberg N, Sieve L. Pregnancy loss, polycystic ovary syndrome, thrombophilia, hypofibrinolysis, enoxaparin, metformin. *Clin Appl Thromb Hemost*. 2004;10(4):323–34.

23. Bodley V, Powers D. Patient with insufficient glandular tissue experiences milk supply increase attributed to progesterone treatment for luteal phase defect. *J Hum Lact*. 1999;15(4):339–43.

24. Betzold C, Hoover K, Snyder C. Delayed lactogenesis II: a comparison of four cases. *J Midwifery Womens Health*. 2004;49(2):132–7.

Chapter 10

1. Uvnäs-Moberg K. Antistress pattern induced by oxytocin. *News Physiol Sci*. 1998;13:22–6.

Neville M. U.S. Department of Health and Human Services. Oxytocin and milk ejection. Available at: http://mammary.nih .gov/reviews/lactation/neville002. Accessed January 12, 2008.

2. Williams N. Maternal psychological issues in the experience of breastfeeding. *J Hum Lact*. 1997;13(1):57–60.

3. Reynolds J. Post traumatic stress disorder after childbirth: the phenomenon of traumatic birth. *CMAJ*. 1997;156(6):831–5.

4. Cowley K. Psychogenic and pharmacologic induction of the let-down reflex can facilitate breastfeeding by tetraplegic women: a report of 3 cases. *Arch Phys Med Rehabil*. 2005;86:1261–4.

5. Feher S, Berger L, Johnson J, Wilde J. Increasing breast milk production for premature infants with a relaxation/imagery audio-tape. *Pediatrics*. 1989;83(1):57–60.

Chapter 11

1. Auerbach K. Sequential and simultaneous breast pumping: a comparison. *Int J Nurs Stud*. 1990;27(3):257–65.

Jones E, Dimmock P, Spencer S. A randomised controlled trial to compare methods of milk expression after preterm delivery. *Arch Dis Child Fetal Neonatal Ed*. 2001;85(2):F91–5.

2. Vallone S. The role of subluxation and chiropractic care in hypolactation. *J Clin Chiropr Pediatr*. 2007;8(1–2):518–24.

3. Jenner C, Filshie J. Galactorrhoea following acupuncture. *Acupunct Med*. 2002;20(2–3):107–8.

Nedkova V, Tanchev S. [The possibilities for stimulating lactation]. *Akush Ginekol (Sofiia)*. 1995;34(2):17–8.

Clavey S. The use of acupuncture for the treatment of insufficient lactation. *Am J Acupunct*. 1996;24(1):35–45.

Sheng P, Xie Q. Relationship between effect of acupuncture on prolactin secretion and central catecholamine and R-aminobutyric acid. *Zhen Ci Yan Jiu*. 1989;14(4):446–51.

Kvist L, Hall-Lord M, Rydhstroem H, Larsson B. A randomised-controlled trial in Sweden of acupuncture and care interventions for the relief of inflammatory symptoms of the breast during lactation. *Midwifery*. 2007;23(2):184–95.

Chapter 12

1. Travers M, Barber M, Tonner E, Quarrie L, Wilde C, Flint D. The role of prolactin and growth hormone in the regulation of casein gene expression and mammary cell survival: relationships to milk synthesis and secretion. *Endocrinology.* 1996;137:1530–9.

2. Speroff L, Glass R, Kase N. *Clinical Gynecologic Endocrinology and Infertility.* 4th ed. Baltimore, MD: Williams & Wilkins; 1989:285.

3. Da Silva O, Knoppert D, Angelini M, Forret P. Effect of domperidone on milk production in mothers of premature newborns: a randomized, double-blind, placebo-controlled trial. *CMAJ.* 2001;164(1):17–21.

4. Gabay M. Galactogogues: medications that induce lactation. *J Hum Lact.* 2002;18(3):274–9.

5. Hale T. *Medications and Mothers' Milk.* 12th ed. Amarillo, TX: Hale Publishing; 2006:277–8.

6. Wan E, Davey K, Page-Sharp M, Hartmann P, Simmer K, Ilett K. Dose-effect study of domperidone as a galactagogue in preterm mothers with insufficient milk supply, and its transfer into milk. *Br J Clin Pharmacol.* 2008 (OnlineEarly article). Available at: http://dx.doi.org/doi:10.1111/j.1365-2125.2008.03207.x. Accessed June 19, 2008.

7. Reddymasu S, Soykan I, McCallum R. Domperidone: review of pharmacology and clinical applications in gastroenterology. *Am J Gastroenterol.* 2007;102(9):2036–45.

Prakash A, Wagstaff A. Domperidone. A review of its use in diabetic gastropathy. *Drugs.* 1998;56(3):429–45.

Soykan I, Sarosiek I, McCallum R. The effect of chronic oral domperidone therapy on gastrointestinal symptoms, gastric emptying, and quality of life in patients with gastroparesis. *Am J Gastroenterol.* 1997;92(6):976–80.

8. Wan E, Davey K, Page-Sharp M, Hartmann P, Simmer K, Ilett K. Dose-effect study of domperidone as a galactagogue in preterm mothers with insufficient milk supply, and its transfer into milk. *Br J Clin Pharmacol.* 2008 (OnlineEarly article). Available at: http://dx.doi.org/doi:10.1111/j.1365-2125.2008.03207.x. Accessed June 19, 2008.

9. Gabay M. Galactogogues: medications that induce lactation. *J Hum Lact.* 2002;18(3):274–9.

Ehrenkrantz R, Ackerman B. Metoclopramide effect on faltering milk production by mothers of premature infants. *Pediatrics.* 1986;78:614.

Kauppila A, Kivinen S, Ylikorkala O. Metoclopramide increases prolactin release and milk secretion in puerperium without stimulating the secretion of thyrotropin and thyroid hormones. *J Clin Endocrinol Metab.* 1981;52(3):436–9.

10. Anfinson T. Akathisia, panic, agoraphobia, and major depression following brief exposure to metoclopramide. *Psychopharmacol Bull.* 2002;36(1):82–93.

Feillet N, Nguyen L, Caillaud D. [Metaclopramide and depression: apropos of a case of a pregnant women]. *Therapie.* 1996;51(5): 600–1.

11. Fisher A, Davis M. Serotonin syndrome caused by selective serotonin reuptake-inhibitors-metoclopramide interaction. *Ann Pharmacother.* 2002;36(1):67–71.

12. Academy of Breastfeeding Medicine. Protocol #9: Use of galactogogues in initiating or augmenting maternal milk supply. Available at: www.bfmed.org/ace-files/protocol/prot9galacto goguesenglish.pdf. Accessed March 7, 2008.

13. Gabbay M, Kelly H. Use of metformin to increase breastmilk production in women with insulin resistance: a case series. Paper presented at: Academy of Breastfeeding Medicine, 8th International Meeting; October 16–20, 2003; Chicago, IL.

14. Jacobson H. *Mother Food: A Breastfeeding Diet Guide with Lactogenic Foods and Herbs—Build Milk Supply, Boost Immunity, Lift Depression, Detox, Lose Weight, Optimize a Baby's IQ, and Reduce Colic and Allergy.* Self-published; 2004.

15. Farnsworth N. Relative safety of herbal medicines. *Herbalgram.* 1993;29:36A–H.

Humphrey S, McKenna D. Herbs and breastfeeding. *Breastfeeding Abstracts.* 1997;17(2):11–2.

16. Saper R, Kales S, Paquin J, et al. Heavy metal content of Ayurvedic herbal medicine products. *JAMA.* 2004;292(23):2868–73.

17. Weed S. *Wise Woman Herbal for the Childbearing Year.* Woodstock, NY: Ash Tree Publishing; 1986:85.

18. Akaogi J, Barker T, Kuroda Y, et al. Role of non-protein amino acid L-canavanine in autoimmunity. *Autoimmun Rev.* 2006;5(6): 429–35.

Alcocer-Varela J, Iglesias A, Llorente L, Alarcón-Segovia D. Effects of L-canavanine on T cells may explain the induction of systemic lupus erythematosus by alfalfa. *Arthritis Rheum.* 1985;28(1):52–7.

Brown A. Lupus erythematosus and nutrition: a review of the literature. *J Ren Nutr.* 2000;10(4):170–83.

19. McGuffin M, Hobbs C, Upton R, Goldberg A, eds. *American Herbal Products Association's Botanical Safety Handbook.* Boca Raton, FL: CRC Press; 1997:21.

20. Foster S. Chaste Tree, Chasteberry—Vitex agnus-castus. Steven Foster Group, Inc. Available at: www.stevenfoster.com/education/monograph/vitex.html. Accessed April 24, 2005.

Upton R. Chaste tree fruit: Vitex agnus-castus: standards of analysis, quality control, and therapeutics. In: *American Herbal Pharmacopoeia and Therapeutic Compendium.* Santa Cruz, CA: American Herbal Pharmacopoeia; 2001.

21. Hoffman D. Herbal medicine materia medica. *HealthWorld* Online. Available at: www.healthy.net/clinic/therapy/herbal/herbic/herbs. Accessed April 24, 2005.

22. Ibid.

23. Javidnia K, Dastgheib L, Mohammadi Samani S, Nasiri A. Antihirsutism activity of fennel (fruits of Foeniculum vulgare) extract. A double-blind placebo controlled study. *Phytomedicine.* 2003;10(6–7):455–8.

24. Swafford S, Berens P. Effect of fenugreek on breast milk volume. *ABM News & Views.* 2000;6(3):21.

Abo El-Nor S. Influence of fenugreek seeds as a galactagogue on milk yield, milk composition and different blood biochemical of lactating buffaloes during midlactation. *Egypt J Dairy Sci.* 1999;27:231–8.

Alamer M, Basiouni G. Feeding effects of fenugreek seeds (Trigonella foenum-graecum L.) on lactation performance, some plasma constituents and growth hormone level in goats. *Pak J Biol Sci.* 2005;8(11):1553–6.

25. Nice F, Coghlan R, Birmingham B. Herbals and breastfeeding. *US Pharm.* 2000;25:28–46.

26. Tahiliani P, Kar A. The combined effects of Trigonella and Allium extracts in the regulation of hyperthyroidism in rats. *Phytomedicine.* 2003;0(8):665–8.

27. Madej A, Persson E, Lundh T, Ridderstråle Y. Thyroid gland function in ovariectomized ewes exposed to phytoestrogens. *J Chromatogr B Analyt Technol Biomed Life Sci.* 2002;777(1–2):281–7.

28. Humphrey S. *The Nursing Mother's Herbal.* Minneapolis, MN: Fairview Press; 2003:320.

29. Fugh-Berman A. "Bust enhancing" herbal products. *Obstet Gynecol.* 2003;101(6):1345–9.

30. Hoffman, D. Herbal medicine materia medica. *HealthWorld* Online. Available at: www.healthy.net/scr/mmedica.asp ?MTId=1&Id=277. Accessed June 16, 2008.

31. McKenna D, Jones K, Hughes K. *Botanical Medicines: The Desk Reference for Major Herbal Supplements.* Binghamton, NY: Haworth Press; 2002.

32. Sabnis P, Gaitonde B, Jetmalani M. Effects of alcoholic extracts of Asparagus racemosus on mammary glands of rats. *Indian J Exp Biol.* 1966;6(1):55–7.

Patel A, Kanitkar U. Asparagus racemosus willd—form bordi, as a galactogogue, in buffaloes. *Indian Vet J.* 1969;46(8):718–21.

33. Sharma S, Ramji S, Kumari S, Bapna J. Randomized controlled trial of Asparagus racemosus (shatavari) as a lactogogue in lactational inadequacy. *Indian Pediatr.* 1996;33(8):675–7.

34. Dalvi S, Nadkarni P, Gupta K. Effect of Asparagus racemosus (shatavari) on gastric emptying time in normal healthy volunteers. *J Postgrad Med.* 1990;36(2):91–4.

Sabnis P, Gaitonde B, Jetmalani M. Effects of alcoholic extracts of Asparagus racemosus on mammary glands of rats. *Indian J Exp Biol.* 1966;6(1):55–7.

35. Goyal R, Singh J, Lal H. *Asparagus racemosus*—an update. *Indian J Med Sci.* 2003;57(9):408–14.

36. Renfrew M, Lang S, Woolridge M. Oxytocin for promoting successful lactation. *Cochrane Database Syst Rev.* 2000;(2): CD000156.

Fewtrell M, Loh K, Blake A, Ridout D, Hawdon J. Randomised, double blind trial of oxytocin nasal spray in mothers expressing breast milk for term infants. *Arch Dis Child Fetal Neonatal Ed.* 2006;91(3):F169–74.

Chapter 14

1. Mohrbacher N. Mothers who chose to pump instead of breast-feeding. *Circle of Caring.* 1996;9(2):1.

2. Cregan M, De Mello T, Kershaw D, McDougall K, Hartmann P. Initiation of lactation in women after preterm birth. *Acta Obstet Gynecol Scand.* 2002;81(9):870–7.

3. Henderson J, Hartmann P, Newnham J, Simmer K. Effect of preterm birth and antenatal corticosteroid treatment on lactogenesis II in women. *Pediatrics.* 2008;121(1):e92–100.

4. Ibid.

5. Chatterton R, Hill P, Aldag J, Hodges K, Belknap S, Zinaman M. Relation of plasma oxytocin and prolactin concentrations to milk production in mothers of preterm infants: influence of stress. *J Clin Endocrinol Metab.* 2000;85(10):3661–8.

6. Hill P, Aldag J, Zinaman M, Chatterton R. Predictors of preterm infant feeding methods and perceived insufficient milk supply at week 12 postpartum. *J Hum Lact.* 2007;23(1):32–8.

Meier P. Expressing milk for your premature baby. Medela. Available at: www.medela.com/for-nursing-mothers/tips-and -solutions/107/expressing-milk-for-your-premature-baby. Accessed January 19, 2008.

7. Gromada K, Spangler A. Breastfeeding twins and higher-order multiples. *J Obstet Gynecol Neonatal Nurs.* 1998;27(4):441–9.

Saint L, Maggiore P, Hartmann P. Yield and nutrient content of milk in eight women breast-feeding twins and one woman breast-feeding triplets. *Br J Nutr.* 1986;56(1):49–58.

8. Hayden T, Thomas C, Forsyth I. Effect of number of young born (litter size) on milk yield of goats: role for placental lactogen. *J Dairy Sci.* 1979;62(1):53–63.

9. Knight C, Sorensen A. Windows in early mammary development: critical or not? *Reproduction.* 2001;122:337–45.

10. Auerbach K, Avery J. Relactation: a study of 366 cases. *Pediatrics.* 1980;65(2):236–42.

11. Jelliffe D, Jelliffe E. Non-puerperal induced lactation. *Pediatrics.* 1972;50(1):170–1.

Auerbach K, Avery J. Induced lactation. A study of adoptive nursing by 240 women. *Am J Dis Child.* 1981;135(4):340–3.

12. Kulski J, Hartmann P, Saint W, Giles P, Gutteridge D. Changes in the milk composition of nonpuerperal women. *Am J Obstet Gynecol.* 1981;139(5):597–604.

13. Hartmann P, Atwood C, Cox D, Daly S. Endocrine and auto-crine strategies for the control of lactation in women and sows. In: Wilde C, Peaker M, Knight D, eds. *Hannah Research Institute Conference on Intercellular Signaling in the Mammary Gland*. New York: Plenum Press; 1994:203–25.

14. Bryant C. Nursing the adopted infant. *J Am Board Fam Med*. 2006;19(4):374–9.

Biervliet F, Maguiness S, Hay D, Killick S, Atkin S. Induction of lactation in the intended mother of a surrogate pregnancy: case report. *Hum Reprod*. 2001;16(3):581–3.

Petraglia F, De Leo V, Sardelli S, Pieroni M, D'Antona N, Genaz-zani A. Domperidone in defective and insufficient lactation. *Eur J Obstet Gynecol Reprod Biol*. 1985;19(5):281–7.

Nemba K. Induced lactation: a study of 37 non-puerperal mothers. *J Trop Pediatr*. 1994;40(4):240–2.

15. Goldfarb L, Newman J. The protocols for induced lactation: a guide for maximizing breastmilk production. Ask Lenore. Available at: www.asklenore.info/breastfeeding/induced_lactation/protocols_intro.html. Accessed January 21, 2008.

Chapter 15

1. Sharma V, Corpse C. Case study revisiting the association between breastfeeding and postpartum depression. *J Hum Lact*. 2008;24(1)77-9.

2. Kendall-Tackett K. *Depression in New Mothers: Causes, Consequences, and Treatment Alternatives*. Binghamton, NY: The Haworth Maltreatment and Trauma Press; 2005:3–4.

Chapter 16

1. Shackleton M, Vaillant F, Simpson K, et al. Generation of a functional mammary gland from a single stem cell. *Nature*. 2006;439(7072):84–8.

Index

About the Authors

Diana West is an International Board Certified Lactation Consultant (IBCLC) in private practice, coauthor with Dr. Elliot Hirsch of *Breastfeeding After Breast and Nipple Procedures*, and author of the *Clinician's Breastfeeding Triage Tool, Defining Your Own Success: Breastfeeding After Breast Reduction Surgery*, as well as numerous magazine articles. She is director of professional development for the International Lactation Consultant's Association board of directors. Diana has a bachelor's degree in psychology, is a retired La Leche League Leader, a website developer, and the administrator of the popular www.bfar.org, www.lowmilksupply.org, www.lactspeak.com, and www.lactask.com websites. She and her family raise German shepherd guide dog puppies for the Seeing Eye. Most important, Diana mothers her three charming, breastfed sons in partnership with her amazing husband, Brad, in their home in the picturesque mountains of western New Jersey.

Lisa Marasco has worked with breastfeeding mothers for more than twenty years, first as a La Leche League Leader and also as an International Board Certified Lactation Consultant (IBCLC) since 1993. She holds a master's degree in human development with specialization in lactation and is recognized for her expertise in milk production problems. Lisa is a contributing author to *Core Curriculum for Lactation Consultant Practice* and continues to research, write, and speak as she pursues answers to milk supply mysteries. She has four adult children and lives with her husband, Tom, in Santa Maria, California, where she continues to help mothers both through her private practice and for Santa Barbara County WIC.